Edited by
BRIAN KIDD
CAMERON STARK

GASKELL

Gaskell is an imprint of the Royal College of Psychiatrists,
17 Belgrave Square, London SW1X 8PG

British Library Cataloguing-in-Publication Data
Management of Violence and Aggression in Health Care
    I. Kidd, Brian II. Stark, Cameron
    III. Burnside, Julia
ISBN 0-902241-84-2

Distributed in North America
by American Psychiatric Press, Inc.
ISBN 0-88048-642-2

Illustrations by Julia Burnside

Printed by Bell & Bain Ltd, Thornliebank, Glasgow

Contents

Contributors

Frances Aiken, SRN, RMN, RNT, DN Cert, BA, MSc(Ethics of Health Care), Cert of IT, Cert in Group Psychotherapy, Lecturer at the Ashworth Training Centre, and Honorary Lecturer at Liverpool University. Formerly a Community Psychiatric Nurse, Ms Aiken is a Project 2000 Tutor, and Facilitator of the University of Liverpool Bachelor of Nursing Mental Health module. She is Chairperson of the Curriculum Development Group for the Diploma in Care in a Controlled Environment.

Glynis Breakwell, BA (Hons), MSc, PhD, MA, CPsychol, FBPsS, Professor of Psychology and Head of Department, University of Surrey. Professor Breakwell's textbooks include *Facing Physical Violence* (1989) and *Managing Violence at Work: Course Leader's Guide and Workbook* (1992 – co-authored with C. Rowett). Twice a member of Council of the British Psychological Society, she is a former Honorary Academic Editor of *The Psychologist*. She was recipient of the British Psychological Society's Myers Award in 1993.

Jeremy Coid, MRCPsych, MPhil, DipCriminol, Senior Lecturer in Forensic Psychiatry, St Bartholomew's Medical College. Dr Coid has published extensively in the fields of violence and psychopathic disorder.

Dilys Jones, BM, MBA, DRCOG, MRCPsych, Medical Director, Special Hospitals Service Authority, London, and Honorary Lecturer in Forensic Psychiatry, Institute of Psychiatry, London. Dr Jones was formerly Senior Medical Officer, Department of Health, where she contributed to the work of the Reed Committee. Dr Jones has also undertaken research on assaults in mental health settings.

Brian Kidd, MB,ChB, MRCPsych, Senior Registrar in Psychiatry, Edith Morgan Centre, Torbay. Dr Kidd has undertaken work on violence to health-care staff, and is currently examining violence towards care workers outside the NHS. He was a founder member of the Multi-Sectoral Interest Group on Violence and Aggression Management Training.

David Leadbetter, BA(Hons), MSc, CQSW, DSW, CSWE, Training and Staff Development Officer, Lothian Regional Council Social Work Department. Research on occupational aggression and co-founder of the Multi Sectoral Interest Group on Violence and Aggression Management and Training. Mr Leadbetter was the co-organiser of the First National Conference on Violence to Staff. He has taught both public sector and voluntary health and welfare agencies and is an accredited Control and Restraint Instructor.

John H. Morgan, BSc Hons, Dip Clin Psychol, CPsychol, Principal Clinical Psychologist, Community Forensic Mental Health Service, St Lawrence's Hospital, Cornwall Health Care Trust. Mr Morgan was formerly Principal Clinical Psychologist at the Broadmoor Hospital.

Margaret C. Orr, MRChB, MRCPsych, Consultant Forensic Psychiatrist and Director of Medical Services, Broadmoor Hospital

Brodie Paterson, RMN, RNMH, RCNT, RNT, BA (Psychol), DipEd, Home Office Registered Control and Restraint Instructor, Lecturer, Forth Valley College of Nursing and Midwifery. Mr Paterson is a member of the Royal College of Nursing's Scottish Board Education and Training Committee and Education and Training Policy Committee.

Erica Robb, BSc, MSc, CPsychol, AFBPS, Head of Tayside Clinical Psychology Forensic Services. Mrs Robb is currently training and offering support to nurses and prison officers who provide peer-group post-incident debriefing to their colleagues following traumatic incidents. This service is being offered to staff at Royal Dundee Liff Hospital and H.M.P. Perth. Mrs Robb was a member of the SHHD Working Party on Alternative Regimes, the SPS Staff Health Care Working Group and the SACRO Bail and Remand Working Party. She is currently a Vice-Chairperson of SACRO.

Cameron Stark, MB,ChB, MPH, MRCPsych, MFPHM, Consultant in Public Health Medicine, Ayrshire and Arran Health Board. Dr Stark is Honorary Secretary of the Multi-Sectoral Interest Group on Violence and Aggression Management Training, and has particular interests in the epidemiology of occupational violence, and the organisational response to violence.

Paul Tarbuck, SRN, RMN, DN, TCert, RNT, BA Theol, ENB 770 Cert, Director of Advanced Nursing Studies and Acting Assistant Director of Nursing Services at Ashworth Hospital, and Honorary Lecturer to Liverpool University. Mr Tarbuck is a member of the English National Board Specialist Panel and Specialist Registry, and an Executive Member of the RCN Society of Mental Health Nursing. He is also a coopted member of the RCN Secure Environments Forum.

Introduction

BRIAN KIDD and CAMERON STARK

Professionals working in the public sector in the United Kingdom report widespread violence towards staff working in areas such as health care, social services and education (Stark & Kidd, 1992). Anecdotal reports suggest that the level may be increasing, as has happened in the USA in the last decade (Davies, 1991). Figures suggest that National Health Service staff have a 1 in 200 chance of major injury through wounding at work, compared with the general public's risk of 1 in 5300 for males and 1 in 25 000 for females (Rowett & Breakwell, 1991).

In health care, concern about increasing violence, along with the fact that there were no national guidelines for employers and staff, led to the Health Services Advisory Committee (HSAC) setting up a working party to examine the extent of the problem. They showed that violence was commonplace in health care and that specific areas, such as accident and emergency, psychiatry and community care carried the highest risk (Health Services Advisory Committee, 1987). They concluded that there was an urgent need for employers and managers to address this issue, by improving the work environment, making appropriate training available to all staff, and supplying adequate facilities for debriefing and post-incident counselling following any violent event.

In social work, Rowett (1986) demonstrated that one in four social workers had been involved in a violent incident, but social work managers appeared to be doing little to reduce the risk to staff (Crane, 1986). At the same time an official inquiry was initiated to investigate the death of a social worker by stabbing (Spokes, 1988). Spokes echoed the HSAC report, making a number of recommendations about training, reporting and environmental improvements.

Violence in mental health settings

Research has repeatedly demonstrated that most assaults in psychiatric hospitals are directed towards nurses or other patients (Noble & Rodger, 1989), and that those nurses most in contact with clients, such as nursing auxiliaries, are the group at highest risk (Rix & Seymour, 1988). American studies, mainly in forensic in-patient units, have estimated injuries to nursing staff at between 16 and 54 per 100 staff per year (Carmel & Hunter, 1989; Hanson & Balk, 1992). Remarkably, Caldwell (1992) found a rate of post-traumatic stress disorder (meeting DSM–III–R criteria; American Psychiatric Association, 1987) in staff of 9% in two American psychiatric units. While this study was hampered by a low response rate and requires replication, it does highlight an important concern. These American results are likely to be overestimates of the situation in the UK. They do, however, demonstrate the size to which the problem can grow in high-risk settings if management is slow to respond.

Whitfield & Shelley (1991) looked at community psychiatric nurses (CPNs) in the UK and found that 8.6% had received a physical injury (from scratches to a stabbing) in the previous 12 months. Verbal abuse was not rated as a serious problem although, as with physical threats, the more CPNs were exposed to this the less seriously they took it. Respondents acknowledged that such incidents raised anxieties about future visits and felt they did not have the training to deal with violence. Forty-six per cent of district health authorities had no operational policy on how to deal with a violent incident, and 60% of CPNs did not know of any guidelines. The authors concluded that few incidents were reported but the subjective effects on staff were great. CPNs felt inadequately trained in managing aggression, and Whitfield & Shelley called for more comprehensive data to be collected from this professional group.

In psychiatry in the UK, 35% of junior doctors in one survey had been assaulted (Kidd & Stark, 1992), similar to the 40% of psychiatric residents in a Canadian study (Chaimowitz & Moscovitch, 1991).

Violence in other settings

General practice

In 1991 Hobbs surveyed over 2000 West Midlands general practitioners (GPs) and, although hampered by a low response rate, found that a quarter of respondents were exposed to violence or aggression from patients. He concluded that violence towards GPs was common and probably increasing, suggesting that improved training in interpersonal skills and aggression management as well as improvements in the running of surgeries might be helpful (Hobbs, 1991). A survey of GPs in London (British Medical Association General Services Committee, 1993), again with a low response rate, found that 43% of those replying had been threatened in the previous two years and 7.6% assaulted (rising to 12% of those with inner-city practices). Myerson (1991) found that 54% of respondents to a similar questionnaire had been involved in a major violent incident, while only 12% had notified the police.

Accident and emergency

Assaults on staff in accident and emergency departments have become increasingly common in the United States (Blank & Mascitti-Mazur, 1991). Schnieden & Marren-Bell (1992) review the situation in the United Kingdom. Assailants are often young men under the influence of alcohol (Cembrowicz & Shepherd, 1992; Pane *et al,* 1991), and up to 20% of incidents occur in waiting rooms (Pane *et al,* 1991). Ambulance staff are also at risk (Tintinalli & McCoy, 1993; *Times,* 1994).

There may be little support for staff (Cembrowicz & Shepherd, 1992), and staff often have little training in how to deal with aggression (Tintinalli & McCoy, 1993). In the United States, physical restraint of aggressive patients is common, and in some cases injuries to patients have resulted in legal action against the hospital (Lavoie *et al,* 1988). The apparent increase in assaults and the vulnerability of hospitals has lead to reviews in the United States with increased security and improved staff training (Brantley, 1992).

Geriatric medicine/psychiatry of old age

A study in Bristol examined the rates of violent incidents in different settings where care was supplied for the elderly (Eastley *et al,* 1993). It was shown that the number of staff assaulted was high (468 assaults on 204 staff in one week), with the staff in hospital caring for those medically unwell and those in the community caring for the mentally ill significantly more likely to be assaulted. Of all the assaults, 87 (19%) were described as "moderate" in severity and 31 staff had required medical treatment or time off work. The authors expressed concern over the lack of trained staff caring for these patients and suggested a need for closer psychogeriatric involvement in homes for the elderly mentally ill.

Employers' responses

These studies carried out by individual professional groups highlight the concern within the caring professions about violence and aggression towards staff. A survey by National Union of Public Employees (NUPE) in 1990 found that 87% of health service staff were very concerned about violence at work (NUPE, 1991). When this was followed up in 1993, the figure had risen to 97% (NUPE, 1994). Other professional groups dealing with the general public, such as teachers and librarians, have also expressed concern over the increase in violence towards their members. This situation, where employers in the health services are effectively failing to meet their obligations, led Glenda Jackson, Labour MP for Hampstead and Highgate, to raise the issue in the House of Commons (Jackson, 1992). In doing so she quoted Lord Skelmersdale, who stated:

> "Provision of a safe workplace is not seen as an accessory but part of the bedrock of service provision. Ignoring this can, if it becomes significantly serious, lead to an inability to maintain that service."

The raising of the issue in Parliament was an important step. It must be remembered, however, that this only arose when a patient and not a staff member was attacked in a hospital.

A multidisciplinary approach

While each profession in the public sector is at risk of increasing violence and some work areas are more dangerous than others, the pattern of violence is remarkably similar across the professions. Those nurses caring for assaultive patients in a secure hospital may be at higher risk. However, librarians in isolated libraries or care staff in an old people's home are also at risk. In such settings the lack of acknowledgement from peers or managers can make the situation intolerable, resulting in poor-quality work or more staff taking time off as a result of ill health. Individual bodies such as unions and professional associations have begun to raise their voices over the lack of direct action from employers. This is to be encouraged. It must not, however, obscure the overall picture, which shows a need for changing attitudes from most (if not all) employers with regard to all of their staff who deal with the public. Exposure to violence is not unique to any professional group and much can be learned from the experience of others.

In Scotland, cooperation among different professions has begun with the emergence of a special interest group of diverse professionals, from doctors, social workers and nurses to prison officers, psychologists and education officers – the Multi-Sectoral Interest Group in Violence and Aggression Management Training (Stark & Kidd, 1992). This forum has allowed sharing of information with regard to available training packages for staff as well as discussion about how to give the issue of violence towards staff a higher exposure in the eyes of the public and the government. It is hoped that by bringing together expertise from many professions a coordinated approach to the needs of staff may be fostered, supported by good-quality multidisciplinary research and evaluation.

There have been many textbooks examining aspects of violence and violence management. Most have been aimed at single professions. All have come from specialists in their respective fields and have thus addressed in detail diverse areas such as the psychological theories behind violence, practical approaches for dealing with the violent client, the medical management of violent psychiatric patients or the assessment of 'dangerousness' by the forensic psychiatrist. Others have described examples of how violence may be encountered at work or have given practical instruction in its management by giving a blow-by-blow account of the moves most likely to be effective when trying to escape or restrain. While these are of value to the staff training officer or aspiring expert, there is a lack of general information on the subject which a professional from any field can use to develop a basic understanding of the problem as it stands for all public service workers. The process of finding information is further hampered by the lack of coordination and availability of research findings, meaning that important work done within one profession may do little to alter the practices of another.

This book attempts to fill this important gap by bringing together the thoughts of prominent workers in the field from the diverse professions which deal with violence and its effects from day to day. (For this reason the term 'client' is generally used in this book to indicate the recipient of care in a variety of settings, and the terms 'professional' or 'practitioner' are used to denote the providers of care and therapy, including members of the medical, nursing, social work and other associated professions and other related groups of practitioners.) It contains chapters on those aspects of violence which must be explored and understood if staff and employers are to work together to reduce the risk of violence to which staff are regularly exposed. It aims to be easily read and practical in its approach – a reference list is provided at the end of each chapter. In a short volume such as this it is impossible to give extensive details. However, each chapter is extensively referenced for those wishing to read further.

References

AMERICAN PSYCHIATRIC ASSOCIATION (1987) *Diagnostic and Statistical Manual of Mental Disorders (3rd edn, revised) (DSM–III–R).* Washington, DC: APA.

BASSE, P. N., JORGENSEN, L. G. & BAK, M.G. (1992) Violence towards personnel of emergency departments. *Ugeskrift for Laeger,* **154,** 1357–1359.

BLANK, C. A. MASCITTI-MAZUR, J. E. (1991) Violence in Philadelphia emergency departments reflects national trends. *Journal of Emergency Nursing,* **17,** 318–321.

BRANTLEY, A. (1992) Rising violence in ERs cause hospitals to redesign security. *Modern Healthcare,* **22,** 44–46.

BRITISH MEDICAL ASSOCIATION GENERAL MEDICAL SERVICES COMMITTEE (1993) *Confidential Survey of London GPs. Final Report.* London: Electoral Reform Ballot Services.

CARMEL, H. & HUNTER, M. (1989) Staff injuries from inpatient violence. *Hospital and Community Psychiatry,* **40,** 41–46.

CEMBROWICZ, G. A. & MOSCOVITCH, A. (1991) Patient assaults on psychiatric residents: the Canadian experience. *Canadian Journal of Psychiatry,* **36,** 107–111.

CRANE, D. (1986) *Violence on Social Workers.* University of East Anglia, Social Work Monograph 46. Norwich: University of East Anglia.

DAVIS, S. (1991) Violence by psychiatric inpatients: a review. *Hospital and Community Psychiatry,* **42,** 585–590.

EASTLEY, R. J., MACPHERSON, R., RICHARDS, H., *et al* (1993) Assaults on professional carers of elderly people. *British Medical Journal,* **307,** 845.

HANSON, R. H. BALK, J. A. (1992) A replication study of staff injuries in a state hospital. *Hospital and Community Psychiatry,* **43,** 836–837.

HEALTH AND SAFETY ADVISORY COMMITTEE (1987) *Violence to Staff.* DHSS Advisory Committee on Violence to Staff Report. London: HMSO.

HOBBS, F. D. R. (1991) Violence in general practice: a survey of general practitioners' views. *British Medical Journal,* **302,** 329–332.

JACKSON, G. (1992) *Hospital Security.* House of Commons official report (Hansard). July 7; 211: col 188 (no. 44).

KIDD, B. & STARK, C. R. (1992) Violence and junior doctors working in psychiatry. *Psychiatric Bulletin of the Royal College of Psychiatrists,* **16,** 144–145.

LAVOIE, F. W., CARTER, G. L., DANZL, D. F., *et al* (1988) Emergency department violence in United States teaching hospitals. *Annals of Emergency Medicine,* **17,** 1227–1233.

Mahoney, B. S. (1991) The extent, nature, and response to victimization of emergency nurses in Pennsylvania. *Journal of Emergency Nursing,* **17,** 282–291.

MYERSON, S. (1991) Violence to general practitioners and fear of violence. *Family Practice,* **8,** 145–147.

NOBLE, P. & RODGER, S. (1989) Violence by Psychiatric in-patients. *British Journal of Psychiatry,* **155,** 384–390.

NATIONAL UNION OF PUBLIC EMPLOYEES (1991) Violence in the NHS. *Health Service News,* 9th April.

—— (1994) *Violence in the Health Service: NUPE Survey.* London: NUPE.

PANE, G. A., VINIARSKI, A. M. & SALNESS, K. A. (1991) Aggression directed toward emergency department staff at a university teaching hospital. *Annals of Emergency Medicine,* **20,** 283–286.

PATERSON, B. & LEADBETTER, D. (1995) Dealing with a hostage situation. *Nursing Times,* **91,** 28–29.

RIX, G. & SEYMOUR, D. (1988) Violent incidents on a regional secure unit. *Journal of Advanced Nursing,* **13,** 746–751.

ROWETT, C. (1986) *Violence in Social Work.* Cambridge: Institute of Criminology.

—— & Breakwell, G. (1992) *Managing Violence at Work.* Windsor: Nelson.

SCHNIEDEN, V. & MARREN-BELL, U. (1992) Violence in the accident and emergency department. *Archives of Emergency Medicine*, **9**, 330–331.

SPOKES, J. (1988) *Report of the Committee of Inquiry into the Care and Aftercare of Miss Sharon Campbell.* London: HMSO.

STARK, C. & KIDD, B. (1992) Violence Management Special Interest Group. *Psychiatric Bulletin*, **16**, 556.

—— & —— (1993) Unite against violence. *British Medical Journal*, **307**, 386.

TIMES (1994) Ambulance crews take the flak in moss side (Anonymous). *Times,* 8th February.

TINTINALLI, J. E. & McCOY, M. (1993) Violent patients and the prehospital provider. [Published erratum appears in *Annals of Emergency Medicine*, **22**, 1635] *Annals of Emergency Medicine*, **22**, 1276–1279.

WHITEFIELD, W. & SHELLEY, P. (1991) Violence and the CPN: a survey. *Community Psychiatric Nursing Journal*, **1**, 13–17.

1 Theories of violence

GLYNIS M. BREAKWELL

Definitions of violence, aggression and assertiveness

It is helpful to start with an attempt to define the terms 'aggressiveness', 'violence' and 'assertiveness'. In everyday conversation, the distinctions between them are often blurred and this can become a disadvantage when deciding how to deal with these three types of behaviour. What they all share is that they involve confrontation. They differ, however, in the form of, and the motivation for, this confrontation.

Assertiveness entails insisting on your rights or opinions. It involves claiming recognition from others that, within the constraints of the law, you have the right to decide how you think, feel and act.

Aggression is typically defined by psychologists as any form of behaviour intended to harm or injure someone against his/her wishes. This means that intentionally harming someone else is not aggression if the injured party wished this to happen. Aggression entails any form of injury, including psychological or emotional injuries. So, for instance, shaming, frightening or threatening can all constitute aggression.

Violence comprises those acts in which there is a deliberate attempt to inflict physical harm. Accidental harm, therefore, does not comprise violence. This distinction between intended and accidental harm is made both in our everyday lives and in the legal system.

Three major psychological explanations of aggression

When explaining aggression or violence, psychologists have usually distinguished two forms: instrumental and emotional.

Instrumental aggression or violence is primarily a means towards some other end. The psychiatrist who is stabbed while a client attempts to steal some psychotropic drug is hurt so that the client

1

might escape, not because the client is angry or upset with the psychiatrist.

Emotional or, as it is sometimes called, angry violence, in contrast, is the deliberate infliction of injury. In this case, doing damage is an end in itself and any instrumental value it has exists purely at a psychological level. A nurse who is attacked when she refuses to administer additional medication is not attacked in order to convince her that she should provide such medication. The attack is driven by anger.

Most of the psychological attempts to explain aggression and violence have focused on the emotional varieties. The other type of violence is felt to be sufficiently explained because of its inherent instrumental value.

There are three main types of psychological explanation: the instinct explanation; the social or cultural learning explanation; and the aversive stimulation explanation (of which the frustration aggression hypothesis represents a special case). These three theories are described briefly in turn.

The instinct explanation

This assumes that aggression is a need. It treats aggression like the need to sleep or eat. It is not learned but is biologically determined and inevitable. If aggression does not occur for some time, the desire for it builds up and eventually it will break out. According to this view, everyone is aggressive and violent, differing only in the ways and situations in which aggression is allowed to be released. Within this framework the aggressive instinct is assumed to have developed because it has survival value.

Such an explanation of aggression, however, has little usefulness for the practitioner because it has little predictive power. It cannot say when aggression will occur, what form it will take, or what interventions are likely to control it. It is impossible to give a realistic example of an aggressive incident which might be exclusively explained by the instinct model. When real incidents are considered it becomes apparent that other explanations must be invoked.

The social or cultural learning explanation

This basically assumes that we are aggressive only because we learn that aggression can be rewarding. By the same token, we can learn not to be aggressive if we find it to be unrewarding or punishing. According to this view aggression is not inevitable. This explanation assumes that aggression and violence are learned behaviours, like all others. Two types of learning are said to be involved: instrumental and observational. Instrumental learning is said to occur when a behaviour is reinforced through rewards and is therefore more likely to recur. Aggressive acts which are rewarded will be produced more frequently. Reward can take many forms. It can be material – for example financial or social rewards such as the awarding of status – or psychological – for example by generating emotional satisfaction. There are many examples of violent incidents where instrumental learning may explain what has occurred.

Case example 1.1

A child is being pushed around by other children. When she is faced with any offence or insult her first action is to hit out. This is commended by her parents, who praise her strongly for standing up for herself.

The child is rewarded for violence in a context demanding self-defence. She will be more likely to exhibit violence in that type of situation subsequently. Moreover, if she continues to be praised for violence, the violent response is likely to generalise (i.e. she will be likely to exhibit violence in similar but not identical situations in the future). For example, she might strike out at a nurse who accidentally hurts her while administering an injection or other treatment. The child will grow to see violence as the appropriate response to any harm done to her, whether intended or not. Such generalisation of learned responses is usually limited by a process of differential reinforcement. Parents who see the child lash out at the nurse are likely to scold or reprimand the child, thus indicating one of the boundaries of appropriate violent self-defence.

Behaviours which result in the removal of something regarded as unpleasant are also reinforced and are likely to recur with increased frequency. For example, a patient who prevents another from bullying her by physical retaliation is likely to use violence as a coping strategy in the future.

While some aggressive behaviours are established through direct reinforcement of this sort, many others are believed to be learned through the observation of others. This is sometimes called social modelling. Bandura (1989) showed that children who watched someone behaving in a violent way would, when subsequently given the opportunity, behave in a similar manner.

There are many studies with adults which also show the results of modelling. While children may learn *how* to be aggressive as a result of watching others, adults appear to learn *when* such behaviour is appropriate in this way. Adults are normally very aware of the social expectations concerning the appropriateness of violence. Their appreciation of these expectations can be changed by watching others in their situation.

Case example 1.2

In a crowded hospital emergency waiting-room a male patient arrives and volubly starts to complain about the waiting time of 45 minutes before he will be seen by a doctor. In spite of attempts to calm him, he becomes more angry and aggressive until, in an attempt to defuse the situation, the charge nurse leads him to a cubicle. At this stage some of the other patients (many of whom have been waiting considerably longer) approach the desk and start to complain angrily about the waiting time. A potentially dangerous situation develops and hospital security have to be called.

The action of the newcomer acts as a learning experience. Observational learning can explain how violent mood or ethos can spread through a collection of unrelated people who just happen to be in the same situation.

One of the advantages of the learning explanation for aggression and violence is that it can explain the existence of cultural and subcultural differences in the amount of violence exhibited. Cultures seem to differ in the amount and types of violence which are available for a child to learn. Anthropological evidence indicates that some societies emphasise the value of pacifism and measure achievement in terms of personal gratification rather than in terms of dominance or power over others. Similarly, sociological evidence proves that subcultures differ greatly in the ways in which they will allow aggression to be expressed. In some, aggression is expected to be expressed physically and in others verbally. Subcultures differ in whom they expect to be aggressive and when. For example, there are differences between the ways men and women are expected to express their aggression. Because people learn from their cultures and subcultures what behaviours are appropriate, the forms of violence and aggression chosen by members of each subculture, as well as the appropriate time to use them, are dictated by norms established within their societies.

This type of explanation of aggression has value for the practitioner because it suggests that, if one knows the norms which control the form, frequency and targets of aggression in a subculture where one works and lives, then one would be better able to predict incidents. It means that the behaviour of individual clients should be analysed in relation to their social background. This is more possible in some practice contexts than in others. It assumes that one already knows something about the individual's background and there are many situations where a practitioner must intervene without having had the opportunity to acquire relevant background information.

The aversive stimulation explanation

This explanation suggests that unpleasant or aversive stimulation increases a person's level of physiological arousal. It is asserted that people are biologically pre-programmed to attempt to avoid heightened arousal, which is experienced as abnormal and unacceptable. Aggression is seen as only one of a range of responses designed to bring about a reduction in arousal levels, largely by eradicating the source of the unpleasant stimulation.

This explanation predicts that aggression may be the preferred response to aversive stimulation under certain circumstances: if other types of response (e.g. avoidance or flight) are impossible – that is, the person is trapped in the situation; if there are clues in the situation which suggest a close association with violent aggression (e.g. the presence of a gun or, in some cultures, types of music, pictures or smells); if the individual has found aggression to be a rewarding solution in the past (e.g. by eliminating the source of an unpleasant stimulation).

The frustration aggression hypothesis is a special example of the aversive stimulation explanation. It was proposed in 1939 and suggested that all aggression was supposed to be preceded by frustration of some sort. Frustration would occur when people could not, for whatever reason, act in a manner which would achieve the goals they had set for themselves. There is considerable evidence that frustration can cause aggression, especially if the frustration is intense or if aggression is seen as likely to result in goal attainment. Frustration does not, however, always result in aggression (e.g. when it is seen to have a justifiable origin) (Berkowitz, 1969).

Frustration is only one sort of unpleasant feeling that people wish to avoid. Physical pain is another, along with noise, crowding or heat. Just as frustration can find alternative expression, so other unpleasant experiences do not necessarily give rise to aggression. Whether they do or not depends on the precise nature of the situation in which they occur, the history of the person involved, and his/her genetic predispositions. So painful experiences can result in avoidance or flight instead of aggression. There is considerable empirical evidence to suggest that painful experiences are most likely to result in aggression if the individual has a history of aggressive responses (particularly if these responses have been effective in gaining rewards), if aggression is likely to eradicate them, or if there are cues for violence prevalent in the situation.

If much aggression and violence can be considered simply as a predictable response to unpleasant experiences, the frequency with which practitioners experience hostility is hardly surprising. Most are, after all, called in precisely when their clients or patients are dealing with events which are unpleasant or distressing.

The situational approach

While each of the three psychological explanations of aggression and violence outlined above have some merit, they are each somewhat unidimensional and inadequate to model the complexities of real violent situations. Real violence takes place against a background of many interacting factors: the social norms of the situation; the social history of the individual; and, not least, the social meanings embedded in the specific situation. The situational approach would argue that most acts of violence are the result of a wide range of interacting factors. These factors are linked with each other and tied to the people involved, the contexts in which they interact and the specific type of interaction which immediately precedes a violent act.

Case example 1.3

A 21-year-old woman walking in the middle of a busy road was picked up by the police and was taken for psychiatric assessment. This was the second occasion that this had occurred, as she had been assessed the previous night under section 136 of the Mental Health Act following a similar incident. On that occasion she had been discharged after 30 minutes, as she was felt to be under stress and not mentally ill. She had a long history of contact with the psychiatric services but had been given a diagnosis of 'personality disorder'. She had often witnessed violent incidents as an in-patient. The psychiatrist knew that she had three children, all of different fathers and all of whom had been taken into care. The woman explained that she was facing eviction by the council after she had thrown stones at her neighbour's children and that she had been deserted by the man with whose child she was now pregnant. The psychiatrist suggested that she might consider an abortion. In response, the woman hit the psychiatrist across the head, shouting "You should know I'm a Catholic!" The doctor later learned that one of the fathers had just gained a residence order for his child, claiming that she was an incapable mother.

Many factors in the history, current life circumstances, psychiatric condition and immediate situation can be seen to be likely to play a part in precipitating her violence. Each of the three major psychological theories could explain her behaviour. However, even taken together, they offer only a broad interpretive framework, and any comprehensive explanation of a violent incident will involve many factors.

Factors associated with the people involved will include their age, education, criminal history, attitudes, socio-economic status, race, mental health, sex and life stress. The context of the interaction will differ in terms of its location, the time of day at which it occurs, the number of people present and the relationships between them and, not least, the geographical or architectural structure of the space in which the interaction occurs. There is no integrative theoretical framework that can be used to explain how all of these factors interact in generating a particular piece of violence at a specific place at a single moment in time.

The advantage of the situational approach for the practitioner lies not in its power to explain, but in its power to direct analysis. It indicates the variety of factors which must be monitored in order to understand how violence operates in practice.

Trigger factors

The situational analysis of violent incidents has led psychologists to suggest that there are trigger factors which can change an interaction between a practitioner and a patient from being potentially violent to actually violent (Breakwell, 1989). The most common trigger factors are:

(a) an intensification of the aversive stimulation (e.g. exacerbation of the experience of pain by insisting that a patient waits an inordinate length of time for treatment)
(b) disinhibition by drugs
(c) the perceived absence of an alternative option to violence
(d) the presence in the situation of cues which reinforce violence (e.g. images depicting violent acts, the presence of a peer group which approves of violence or the use of words or phrases – known as 'barbs' – which are provocative to the person concerned)
(e) the experience of sudden major life changes or the advent of new stressors
(f) attempts to interpret the individual's behaviour as psychotic when he/she regards it as normal

The assault cycle

Situational analyses of acts of violence have resulted in researchers asserting that an act of violence is part of a cycle of behaviour – the assault cycle (Fig. 1.1.). The structure of the assault cycle was first described by Paul Smith, staff trainer for the Californian State Department of Corrective Services. He analysed hundreds of accounts of violent incidents and identified a series of inter-related phases typically found in most assault situations (for details see Kaplan & Wheeler, 1983).

The trigger phase

Irrespective of setting, people have a normal baseline set of behaviours and for almost everyone this normal behaviour is non-aggressive most of the time. The triggering phase is the point at which the individual first indicates a movement away from his/her normal behaviour. Such changes may be perceived in verbal or non-verbal behaviour. The less detailed understanding the staff has of any individual the more easily can these early warning signs be missed.

The escalation phase

This phase leads directly to violent behaviour. The individual's behaviour deviates more and more from baseline levels. If there is no intervention, the deviation becomes both increasingly more obvious and less amenable to diversion. The individual is likely to become overly focused on a particular issue and is less likely to

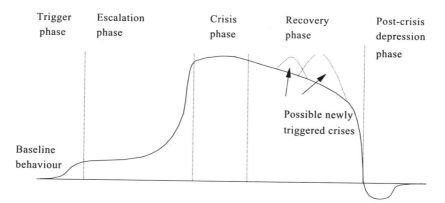

Fig. 1.1. Phases of a typical assault cycle (adapted from Rowett & Breakwell, 1992)

respond to any form of rational intervention. It is therefore important to intervene as early as possible in this phase by, for example, counselling, removing the client from the environment, supplying an alternative task or using anger-management techniques.

The crisis phase

As the individual becomes increasingly physically, emotionally and psychologically aroused, control over aggressive impulses lessens and actual violent behaviour becomes more likely. In this phase, the least effective strategy is to adopt an intervention which presumes that the individual can respond rationally. Once the crisis phase has been reached, it is advisable to focus on the safety of anyone under threat. Options may be very limited – escape, physical restraint, seeking help from others or physical protection by the imposition of barriers (e.g. doors, desks).

The recovery phase

The individual will gradually return to normal baseline behaviour once the violent act has occurred. It is at this point that most errors of intervention occur. The high state of physical and emotional arousal can remain for up to one and a half hours after the incident itself. Attempts at intervention in this period can result in the renewal of the attack. In fact, it appears that, during the recovery phase, the individual is particularly sensitive to the trigger factors described earlier.

Post-crisis depression phase

In this phase the individual often regresses below normal baseline behaviour. Mental and physical exhaustion is common and the individual may become tearful, remorseful, guilty, ashamed, distraught or despairing. The crisis is over and the individual may be receptive to interventions designed to relieve guilt, understand the incident and prevent recurrence.

The victim's experience of the assault cycle

In the descriptions above, the phases of the assault cycle have been depicted in terms of its experience on the part of the aggressor. It should be emphasised that there is evidence to support the argument that the individual having to deal with the potential aggressor (often the potential victim) experiences a similar set of phases during the cycle. During the escalation phase the potential victim has a considerable increase in arousal which peaks during the crisis phase. This means that at precisely the moment when it is important for the potential victim to behave in a rational and effective manner he/she is likely to be working with a reduced capacity. The heightening of physical and psychological arousal is likely to hamper the practitioner's control and effectiveness. During the recovery phase, the practitioner is similarly likely to echo the experiences of the aggressor, being easily tipped into excessive anxiety or even hilarity as a result. In the post-crisis depression phase the practitioner will feel parallel exhaustion or fatigue to that of the aggressor. It is therefore difficult for the practitioner/victim to cope with the organisation and provision of the interventions necessary for the client/aggressor at this stage.

Intervening in the cycle

The assault cycle is a useful tool for schematising a process which occurs during a typical episode of aggressive behaviour. The analysis emphasises that intervention is possible at all times except in the crisis phase, where practitioners should primarily consider aspects of safety for themselves and the client. Both the aggressor and victim experience high levels of physical and psychological arousal which affects how they both behave. The practitioner must be aware of this and develop ways to overcome it.

Finally, the analysis suggests that most violent incidents are understandable and can be prevented or at least ameliorated with the correct interventions at the appropriate time.

References

BANDURA, A. (1989) Perceived self-efficacy in the exercise of personal agency. *Psychologist*, **2**, 411–424.

BERKOWITZ, L. (ed.) (1969) *Roots of Aggression: A Re-examination of the Frustration-Aggression Hypothesis*. New York: Atherton.

BREAKWELL, G. M. (1989) *Facing Physical Violence*. London: British Psychological Society/Routledge.

KAPLAN, S. G. & WHEELER, E. G. (1983) Survival skills for working with potentially violent clients. *Social Casework*, **64**, 339–374.

ROWETT, C. & BREAKWELL, G. M. (1992) *Managing Violence at Work*. Slough: NFER-Nelson.

Summary points

- Assertiveness, aggression and violence all involve confrontation, although the form of and motivation for the confrontation differs.
- Aggression is any behaviour intended to harm people against their wishes and includes psychological and emotional injury.
- Violence deliberately attempts to inflict physical harm.
- Psychologists describe two forms of aggression/violence: instrumental – a means to an end; and emotional – deliberately inflicting injury.
- Psychologists have three main explanations for aggression/violence: instinct – aggression is a basic need; social/cultural learning – it is learned that violence brings rewards; aversive stimulation – aggression is used to avoid states of heightened arousal.
- It is likely that all three explanations are important and any situation is an interplay of many factors related to the individuals concerned and the situation they are in – the situational approach.
- Trigger factors can trigger actual violence in a potential aggressor.
- The assault cycle describes the five phases of any violent incident. The action which can be taken depends on the phase of the cycle the aggressor is in. The victim goes through similar phases. (Phase-specific responses are discussed in greater detail in Chapter 4.)

2 Prediction of dangerousness

DILYS JONES

Some people show characteristics which may make them more likely to assault. Easier identification of the dangerous patient is likely to help staff in any setting to be more aware and to deal with these people more safely.

In the field of mental illness, the forensic psychiatrist has an important role in the assessment of the potential dangerousness of a person. This chapter examines the concept of dangerousness from the perspective of the forensic psychiatrist. It examines the usefulness of this concept within normal work practices as well as the many difficulties experienced when trying to predict violence. Although the perspective of forensic psychiatry may appear limiting, the principles will be relevant to others working with potentially violent individuals. The role of Special Hospitals is discussed as many professionals will have contact with patients who have passed through the Special Hospital system. In addition, it is helpful for workers in all agencies to be familiar with the psychiatric concept of dangerousness, and the evidence on which the concept is based.

It has been said that psychiatrists are no more able to predict dangerousness than anyone else. This is an area of some debate and may be examined alongside studies of reoffending among those discharged from Special Hospitals. Recently there has been considerable concern about some patients who, when discharged from general psychiatric hospitals, have killed. This has resulted in the establishment of a confidential enquiry by the Royal College of Psychiatrists and also the announcement of new proposals by the Secretary of State for Health to increase the supervision of some patients in the community after discharge from hospital.

Definition of dangerousness

Although important decisions are based on it, there is no consensus on the meaning of the term 'dangerousness'. Scott (1977) defined it as "an unpredictable and untreatable tendency to inflict or risk serious, irreversible injury or destruction, or to induce others to do so". Faulk (1988), however, points out that others have objected to the use of "unpredictable and untreatable", because the recognition of risk or the treatability of the injury does not reduce the danger, although it does allow protective steps to be taken. The *Collins English Dictionary* (3rd edn, 1979) defines danger as "a person or thing that may cause injury, pain, etc." and being in danger as "the state of being vulnerable to injury, loss or evil; risk". The Butler Committee (Home Office and Department of Health and Social Security, 1975) equated 'dangerousness' with "a propensity to cause serious physical injury or lasting physical harm". The Reed Committee stated:

> "It is evident that there are widely varying forms and levels of dangerousness as regards both the clinical condition of the individual concerned and the circumstances in which the individual finds himself at any particular time. But the issue of dangerousness and of the means of assessing and predicting its incidence in individual cases in a consistent and objective way is central to the work of forensic psychiatry." (Review of Health and Social Services for Mentally Disordered Offenders and Others Requiring Similar Services, 1992)

Others use the term to mean the risk of inflicting serious violence on others, causing serious psychological harm, and damaging property where there is a risk of physical injury to others. The inclusion of psychological harm is important, as this can be the effect of some crimes where there is no physical injury.

Gunn (1982) describes his understanding of the term as being of three elements – destructiveness, prediction and fear. The latter, he says, makes it at least partially subjective and it can therefore never be entirely objective. Dangerousness does not have the characteristics of a finite measurement like weight, length or speed. It is essentially an opinion which is made taking into account all views and information about an individual, and it will be affected by the previous experience or knowledge of the psychiatric team.

The difficulty in defining the concept of dangerousness and the discovery that it cannot be measured cast doubt on whether or not it is of any practical use. It is certainly important in the sense that psychiatrists will be asked questions about it by the authorities and will need to consider it in their day-to-day management of their patients. Whether or not they are the appropriate or best-equipped professionals to do this is discussed below, but there is no doubt that they currently have to do it and must therefore strive to do it to the best of their abilities, using whatever tools are available to them.

The psychiatrist may be requested to give an opinion on how a person will behave in a new and less secure setting or may advise a mental health review tribunal, magistrate, judge at court or colleagues in other parts of the psychiatric services. They may also advise C3 Division at the Home Office as well as making a report to the Advisory Board (in the case of a patient) or to the parole board (in the case of a prisoner). Assessment of dangerousness has to take into account the factors which would be therapeutically beneficial to management and weigh them against the need for security in order to protect the safety of the public, the patient, other people and staff. It has to take into account the history, the individual's characteristics, how well his/her mental disorder is responding to treatment, the nature of the therapeutic alliance between the clinical team and the patient and the environment in which they are likely to interact.

In real terms, the psychiatrist is looking at a hierarchical structure of practice in the sense that recommendations following assessment of dangerousness are designed to prevent dangerous behaviour. However, if a sequence of events is observed to be in motion which might lead to dangerous behaviour, there are ways of de-escalating or defusing this. Finally, where violent incidents have occurred, there are methods of damage limitation (tertiary prevention) which must be put into operation. Some of these issues are discussed further in Chapter 4.

The assessment of risk

Although dangerousness is a term used frequently in clinical practice, in order to make clinical decisions, the forensic psychiatrist uses the prediction of dangerousness in the context of an assessment of the risk of a person exhibiting such behaviour in a particular environment or situation. A number of problems have arisen here. Research (Cocozza & Steadman, 1978) has shown that the clinical predictions made are rather inaccurate. Monahan (1988) outlines how even when performing optimally, psychiatrists considerably overpredict the likelihood of violent behaviour.

The main practical method for the assessment of risk posed by an individual focuses on the *clinical approach* (Scott, 1977; Faulk, 1988).

This involves taking a full history, including information from family, friends and carers, and being assiduous in the collection of information about the patient and the offending behaviour. The *actuarial approach*, on the other hand, involves the assessment of risk based on statistics and population studies (Carson, 1990; Clark *et al*, 1993). Others have attempted to measure dangerousness, or aspects of it, using research indices or rating scales (Menzies *et al*, 1985; Heilbrun, 1990).

It is widely recognised that, despite some progress in the latter approaches, the clinician is faced with "imperfect technology" (Heilbrun, 1990). As Faulk (1988) notes, the "current situation remains that the clinician must continue to try to make an assessment of dangerousness of mentally disordered offenders and in doing so, has to rely on criteria which have not been tested scientifically".

Each of the approaches noted above complements the other and they are best used together. As Snowden (1993) says, however:

> "We cannot practice forensic psychiatry by taking no risks neither should we take risks without a sound knowledge base to guide us . . . .The time has now come for forensic psychiatry to adopt a more logical and rational approach to both decision-making and risk-taking."

The clinical approach

Scott (1977) states that it is "patience, thoroughness and persistence" in the process of information gathering, "rather than any diagnostic or interviewing brilliance," that provides the surest approach in the assessment of dangerousness.

In the first instance, Special Hospital forensic psychiatrists will often find themselves in the position of providing an opinion as to whether or not a person should be treated in the Special Hospital rather than in another facility with less security (e.g. a general psychiatric unit) or in prison. Meeting the criteria for the presence of mental disorder (and treatability or prevention of deterioration) is necessary for all individuals when considering detaining patients for treatment under the Mental Health Act 1983. (See Chapter 5 for details of the Mental Health Acts.) The specific issue when deciding whether a patient needs admission to a Special Hospital as opposed to one which is less secure is dangerousness. The National Health Service Act 1977 requires Special Hospitals to provide treatment of individuals under conditions of special security on account of their dangerous, violent or criminal propensities. The person has to be "a grave and immediate risk to others".

First, a full history is taken, including family history, personal history, psychiatric history, offending history, sexual history and examination of mental state. In particular, while gathering this information, the psychiatrist should try:

(a) to identify precipitants for the offending behaviour, the capacity for patients to understand what they have done, their ability to empathise with victims and whether or not there is any potential for developing a therapeutic alliance

(b) to determine whether patients have learnt from their behaviour and whether they have been cooperative with a treatment regimen in the past

(c) to know how patients have coped in a hospital setting and how they have responded to it (have they absconded or tried to abscond?)

(d) to determine whether there is a recurring behaviour pattern or whether a pattern of escalation with greater dangerousness in the offending behaviour is being exhibited on each occasion.

The precise offence itself is not an indication of dangerousness *per se* (Scott, 1977) but the nature of the behaviour leading to the offence, the nature of the offence itself, and its circumstances should be determined. The use or manufacture of weapons is of importance. Dangerous and violent behaviour is confined to a small proportion of the population and is viewed as socially unacceptable (except in special circumstances such as during wartime). Many authors refer to the need to examine carefully the factors which have led to the "crossing of the threshold into dangerous behaviour" (Scott, 1977) and which often provide the key to understanding the individual's actions. Scott also notes the importance of being assiduous in the collection of data relating to past records, the checking of information against other sources and talking to others, such as the probation officer, who will also report to a court and will have valuable knowledge of the individual. This includes examining the depositions and witness statements relating to the index offence.

The multidisciplinary approach is important and although tight time schedules may sometimes dictate against it, the opinions of the psychologist and psychiatric nurse are invaluable. This is particularly so in relation to possible behavioural aspects of a future treatment programme, psychological aspects of risk assessment, and how a potential patient might fit into the proposed therapeutic environment, with particular respect to any dangers that the environment might present with reference to the person being assessed.

During the assessment it will usually be possible to collect together sufficient information to form an opinion about dangerousness or at the very least to determine what level of security would be required in order safely to assess treatability further, if that were the appropriate approach. It will also provide other 'leads' for information, such as school reports if, for example, the individual has had special schooling. These need to be followed up thoroughly and often swiftly.

With reference to assessment of risk of individuals who are subject to restriction orders (see Chapter 5), the recommendations of clinicians are reviewed by the Home Secretary, aided by C3 Division at the Home Office. (This process is different in Scotland.) This is in relation to permission for escorted rehabilitation trips outside the hospital, unescorted leave outside the hospital, and decisions relating to trial leave, transfer and discharge of the patient. The Home Secretary has a primary role in preserving public safety (Pickersgill, 1990). (See Appendices to Chapter 5.)

The actuarial approach

This is risk assessment based on the use of statistical data. It is an approach which should be used to enhance the clinical assessments made on the basis of the multidisciplinary view of the patient and an examination of the records (Dowie, 1990). For example, research (Quinsey *et al*, 1975; Bailey & MacCulloch, 1992*a,b*) has examined reconviction rates for those discharged under different conditions. It suggests that reconviction rates are higher for patients discharged into the community directly from Special Hospitals than for those initially transferred to a lower-security facility. This is also the case for those who are on a conditional discharge from their restriction order rather than those on an absolute discharge. Numbers of previous serious offences are seen to be associated with higher rates of reconviction for violent offences. As stated by Owens & Schoenfeldt (1979), past behaviour is the best predictor of future behaviour. This is particularly so with respect to the type and frequency of previous convictions (Hill, 1985; Farrington & West, 1990).

Bailey & MacCulloch (1992*a,b*) found that, of those discharged from the Special Hospital, there were greater reconviction rates for those with psychopathic disorder than for those with mental illness. Almost all the first reconvictions for those with mental illness occurred in the first two and a half years after discharge, whereas for those with psychopathic disorder, reconvictions often occurred well beyond this period. Overall, 75% of those with psychopathic disorder and 90% of the mentally ill did not reoffend seriously. Bailey

& MacCulloch made the point that very many more of these studies are required, using information technology to collect and collate the data. One of the uses of such data is that they highlight some groups as being more dangerous than others, for example those with psychopathic disorder being more likely to reoffend after discharge. This can help the clinician in estimating risk related to individuals, provided that the statistical information is used as an adjunct to the clinical assessment.

There are similar, older studies. In 1966, a patient called Johnnie K. Baxstrom won his case in the Supreme Court of the United States. It upheld his claim that he had been denied equal protection of the laws of the statutory procedure under which he was then being held at the Dannemara State Hospital. He was being detained in hospital (having been sent there from prison) after his prison sentence expired. Following the court decision nearly a thousand individuals in a similar position were transferred from New York State maximum-security hospitals to ordinary psychiatric hospitals and were subsequently discharged into the community. They had been in prison or hospital for an average of 18 years.

After discharge they were followed up. Cocozza & Steadman (1975, 1978) found that 15% had shown violent assaultiveness against people. They also found that, of the whole 920 men transferred, three committed homicide within four years of release. The majority presented no such problems and the point was made that many had been kept in high-security facilities much longer than had been necessary. This again raised the issue of the degree of accuracy psychiatrists have when they make predictions about dangerousness. This study illustrates the high level of false positives.

Clinical decision making

Scott (1977) makes the point that risk assessment should be continuous, that is a dynamic and reiterative process over time. Snowden (1993) is keen for such decision making to be more rigorous and for it to be more thoroughly audited. He and others have pointed out the need to protect the public and therefore to ensure that our clinical decision-making is as good as it can be given our current state of knowledge (Review of Procedures for the Discharge and Supervision of Psychiatric Patients and Subject to Special Restrictions, 1973). There is a clear need to improve it and this includes the need to develop standardised procedures for supporting the decision-making process. As Dowie & Elstein (1988) state, "Clinicians have traditionally held clinical judgement and decision making in high regard and been suspicious of attempts to explore them systematically with a view to making explicit their precise character". We are perhaps fortunate within the Special Hospitals Service in that the Special Hospitals Service Authority is currently developing support systems for clinical decision making. As it cares for some of the most potentially dangerous people, it is very appropriate that the Special Hospitals Service is at the forefront of such activity. It is likely, however, that this approach will also be of value to clinicians working in non-secure settings.

From the perspective of the patient it is also important that professionals strive to ensure that clinical decision making is as accurate as possible. As with the Baxstrom cases, it is an injustice to detain anyone within a high-security hospital for any longer than he/she needs to be there. Advice to the Home Secretary and to the mental health review tribunals in the case of restricted patients is therefore very important. Both have the power to discharge those detained either conditionally or absolutely. Similarly, it will lead clinicians to begin to ask questions about, and to develop research relating to whether there are, common factors found within the clinical decision-making process which may be predictive of relapse or reoffending, but which have not yet been sufficiently clarified.

MacCulloch & Bailey (1993) define levels of security with reference to leaving Special Hospitals. They state that in one sense levels of security mirror perceived dangerousness. "Descriptions of levels of security must contain three elements: physical structure; dynamic or interactive security provided by the clinical staff" and "the patient's control of his own behaviour". They point out the need for a continuum of care for mentally disordered offenders, which commences in maximum security and ends with living in the community. A major part of assessing dangerousness is careful observation with regard to how a person settles into a new environment and how he/she copes with increased personal responsibility and freedom. It is often the case that this is a time which can prove very unsettling and when, under stress, the patient can relapse into psychosis or return to old, potentially dangerous, patterns of behaviour.

Mental illness and dangerousness

Throughout history the mentally ill have been regarded as more prone to violent behaviour than the rest of the population and it was not until recently that much research was carried out in this area. The factors causing violence are many and varied. As Gunn (1991) stated, "Violence is universal in the animal kingdom. Perhaps it has biological advantages." He described how it may create the hierarchies and sanctions of social life in the animal kingdom. Gunn (1991) and Faulk (1988) outlined three theories of violence: the instinct hypothesis; the frustration hypothesis and the social learning/learned response hypothesis. However, it is widely accepted that violence is a multifactorial phenomenon and with reference to the human race it has not been shown to be associated with any particular ethnic group (Mann, 1993). The theoretical background is discussed in greater detail in Chapter 1.

It is clear that for some people who become mentally ill and perpetuate violent behaviour or offences the violence is related directly to their mental illness.

Case example 2.1

A patient with schizophrenia held the delusional belief that members of the nursing staff were being programmed by the television set to spy on him and that eventually they would harm him if he did not harm them first. This belief led to attacks on staff members.

For others with mental illness there may not be such a clear link between their illness and violent behaviour. For some, with an additional diagnosis of a personality disorder as well as mental illness, there may be a subtle interaction of a number of factors, including both diagnoses and a particular set of circumstances, with drug or alcohol misuse often serving to disinhibit the perpetrator further, making violent offending behaviour more likely. Feldmann *et al* (1990) noted the possibility of cofactors precipitating or eliciting events, particularly when the perpetrator had a personality disorder.

Taylor & Gunn (1984) examined the risk of violence among psychotic men. They reviewed the case records of a sample of 1241 men remanded to Brixton Prison over a four-month period. Of the total intake of 2743 men over that period, 8.7% were psychotic, 70% of whom suffered from schizophrenia. Of this group, they found that the risk of violence was high – 9% of non-fatal personal assaults and 21% of offences relating to damage. They found a higher prevalence of schizophrenia among those convicted of homicide (11% of 0.1–0.4%) than was expected when compared with the local population in Greater London.

Hafner & Boker (1973) examined violent offending among the mentally abnormal over the course of a decade in West Germany. They concluded that this group had no greater likelihood of committing violent acts than the general population. However, they included under the term 'mentally abnormal' people with depression, organic brain syndrome and mental handicap as well as schizophrenia. If the results for the latter diagnostic group are taken from their study, Hafner & Boker also showed people with schizophrenia to have a higher than expected rate of violent offending, while the other diagnostic groups had a lower than expected rate. They found that people with schizophrenia who were violent shared many of their demographic characteristics with those who were violent from the general population. They had the same intelligence and educational levels and most were men.

Violent incidents in hospitals – predicting the risk

The majority of research carried out by psychiatrists in this area has been in the USA (e.g. Madden *et al*, 1976; Tardiff, 1983; Ionno, 1983). Some, however, has been performed in the UK (e.g. Fottrell, 1980; Edwards *et al*, 1988).

The rate of assaults in hospitals in the UK is much lower than in the USA. A survey carried out by the Health and Safety Advisory Committee (1987) showed that 26.8% of staff in psychiatric facilities had been assaulted by patients, receiving minor injuries, with 1.6% receiving more serious injuries. Edwards *et al* (1988) found an assault rate of 0.39 assaults/bed/year in an English psychiatric unit as compared with 1.36 assaults/bed/year in 14 North American psychiatric units. Other surveys have published data in terms of assault rates but the results are not comparable because of the different definitions of 'assault'.

Fottrell (1980) and Edwards *et al* (1988) showed that assaults can occur at almost any time of the day, although most occur in the mornings, at times when clients' activities are often unstructured. Other work has suggested that the environment plays a part – the noise level and overcrowding are significant factors, as is the temperature and the way in which the individual is being managed. As in all patient–professional interactions, skilled and sensitive handling is of the essence. Research has also shown provocation to be a factor in many assaults, emphasising the importance of a non-confrontational approach.

The majority of violent incidents in psychiatric hospitals are not serious (Fottrell, 1978; Edwards *et al*, 1988). A small number of individuals are responsible for a large number of assaults. Fottrell (1978) found that this minority repeatedly behaved in this fashion. He noted the need to know more about how a number of factors possibly interacted in leading to violent incidents, including "overcrowding, understaffing, poor staff–patient relationships and inadequate therapeutic atmosphere". Hodgkinson *et al* (1985) found that violent incidents occurred most frequently during the busiest period on the ward – that is between 7 a.m. and 12 noon. Ruben *et al* (1980) examined physical attacks on psychiatric residents at a Los Angeles hospital and found that most incidents occurred "during or after an incident in which the residents had frustrated the patient in some way". They also found that the personality of the psychiatrist was related to being attacked, with those who were "highly irritable, who speak up when mildly angry and who are likely to fight when faced with a physically threatening situation are subsequently more likely to be attacked than psychiatrists who do not have these attributes". Hodgkinson *et al* (1985) found that, while 65% of staff who were assaulted were involved in only one incident, 5% were involved in 20% of incidents. They noted that many of this group who were repeatedly assaulted worked in high-risk areas. However, they also thought it possible that "the element of the individuals' preferred management style of certain situations" may well have contributed to their being more frequently assaulted.

Although fatal assaults by patients on care workers are more common in the USA (Bernstein, 1981; Annis & Baker, 1986), such assaults are not unkown in the UK (Department of Health and Social Security, 1988).

With reference to predicting which patients are likely to become violent in hospital, a North American study by Werner *et al* (1984) asked 15 psychiatrists to review 40 male in-patients on the psychiatric intensive-care unit. Violence was predicted by the psychiatrists if hostility, agitation, previous assaultiveness or suspiciousness were present. However, this left unidentified a group who had been violent, but had exhibited hypervigilance, engagement and attentiveness and were experiencing hallucinations. The authors concluded that potentially assaultive individuals do not necessarily fit any particular pattern. The importance of control in interviewing every patient is emphasised in Chapter 3.

Management of the potentially dangerous patient – on the ward and at interview

The key to the management of the potentially dangerous patient has been described by Faulk (1988) and Scott (1977). It is essential to strive for a therapeutic alliance between the patient and the clinical team, in which patients can feel safe and secure and feel that their needs have been acknowledged and are seen as important. Clearly, this may be difficult to achieve initially, particularly if the patient is floridly psychotic or has had past negative experiences. The importance of a non-confrontational approach while developing such a rapport cannot be over-emphasised in the successful prevention of violence or when evaluating the risk of violence. All professional staff need appropriate training in these areas. Staff must feel confident and be equipped with the appropriate skills. (See Chapter 4 for further details.)

It is important that members of the clinical team know their patients well and can respond quickly to any worrying observations of behavioural change which could indicate a breakdown of communication or be a prelude to disturbed behaviour.

Once the patient is familiar to staff it is often clear that there is a pattern of behaviour which precedes violence.

Case example 2.1 (*continued*)

The patient with schizophrenia who believed staff were plotting against him showed a number of early signs before any incident. He would initially become withdrawn and would appear to be experiencing auditory hallucinations (smiling inappropriately, 'talking' to his voices). This would be followed by his missing meals and not attending to his personal hygiene. He would then become frankly deluded (i.e. develop his beliefs about the staff plotting against him) and this would lead to assaultive behaviour. It was impossible to establish a therapeutic rapport on admission. However, this became possible as his symptoms responded to treatment. The preventive approach involved developing the therapeutic relationship sufficiently for the patient to be able to trust the clinical team so that he could divulge his psychotic experiences. With time and an increasing knowledge of the patient, he was able to tell staff when he became more unwell and staff were able to help him develop a greater awareness and insight into his condition and to relate the worsening of his symptoms to episodes of stress in his life.

It is by such a relationship being present that it is possible to gain access to the client's inner world and by doing so to be less at risk of being taken by surprise by his behaviour. It may also be possible to help him understand and come to terms with the nature of his offence. Often the pattern of behaviour leading to the offence may be seen again within the hospital. This provides an excellent opportunity to help the patient develop a better understanding of himself and, therefore, to become potentially 'safer'. When this is not possible an individual must be regarded as being a greater 'risk'.

In order to make the greatest use of these opportunities, members of the clinical team must know their patient well individually and

Summary points

- Dangerousness is difficult to define and measure objectively.
- Assessment of risk in as consistent and objective a way as possible is a central function of the forensic psychiatrist.
- The assessment weighs up issues for the individual (freedom etc.) against public safety and the safety of the individuals.
- Assessment of risk ideally takes both a clinical approach (based on information regarding an individual) and an actuarial approach (based on statistics and population studies).
- Predictors of violence can be inaccurate and psychiatrists tend to overpredict violent behaviour.
- Previous behaviour is the best predictor of future behaviour.
- The degree of dangerousness changes with internal characteristics of the client (e.g. mental illness) and external (environmental) influences.

collectively. The sharing of information by the clinical team is of the essence in creating a rich database on which to form an effective treatment programme. The dynamics of the clinical team are therefore of fundamental importance. Each member is an equal; the consultant psychiatrist may chair the clinical team meetings, but it will probably be the nursing assistant who has been told the most important piece of information by the patient about him-/herself. Those who are with patients most can provide the best description of their behaviour and offer the best clues about why they behave as they do. Management programmes and other interventions can then be applied proactively to influence unwanted behaviour. The clinical team meeting is the vehicle or forum for the consideration of dangerousness. It is here that all aspects of a client's care and progress will be analysed and recommendations made about his/her future. Important factors for such activity to be effective therefore include appropriate training, effective communication and sharing of information, a high regard by individual team members for each other and appropriate emphasis on the value of individual contributions.

References

ANNIS, L. V. & BAKER, C. A. (1986) A psychiatrist's murder in a mental hospital. *Hospital and Community Psychiatry*, **37**, 505–506.

BERNSTEIN, H. A. (1981) Survey of threats and assaults directed towards psychotherapists. *American Journal of Psychotherapy*, **35**, 542–549.

BAILEY, J. & MacCULLOCH, M. (1992*a*) Characteristics of 112 cases discharged directly to the community from a new special hospital and some comparisons of performance. *Journal of Forensic Psychiatry*, **3**, 91–112.

—— & —— (1992*b*) Patterns of reconviction in patients discharged directly to the community from a special hospital: implications for after-care. *Journal of Forensic Psychiatry*, **3**, 445–461.

CARSON, D. (ed.) (1990) *Risk Taking in Mental Disorder*. England: SLE Publication.

CLARK, D. A., FISHER, M. J. & McDOUGALL, C. (1993) A new methodology for assessing the level of risk in incarcerated offenders. *British Journal of Criminology*, **33**, 436–448.

COCOZZA, J. J. & STEADMAN, H. J. (1978) *Predictions in Psychiatry: An Example of Misplaced Confidence in Experts*. Berkeley: University of California Press.

DOWIE, J. (1990) Clinical decision making. Risk is a dangerous word and hubris is a sin. In *Risk Taking in Mental Disorder* (ed. D. Carson). pp 28–39. England: SLE Publication.

—— & ELSTEIN, E. (eds) (1988) *Professional Judgement: A Reader in Clinical Decision Making*. Cambridge: Cambridge University Press.

DEPARTMENT OF HEALTH (1993) *Legislation Planned to Provide for Supervised Discharge of Psychiatric Patients*, H93/908. Press release, 12 August. London: DoH.

DEPARTMENT OF HEALTH AND SOCIAL SECURITY (1988) *Report of the Committee of Enquiry into the Care and After-care of Miss Sharon Campbell*. Chairman John Spokes QC. London: HMSO CM 440.

EDWARDS, J. G., JONES, D., REID, W. H., *et al* (1988) Physical assaults in a psychiatric unit of a general hospital. *American Journal of Psychiatry*, **145**, 1368–1371.

FARRINGTON, D. P. & WEST, D. J. (1990) The Cambridge study in delinquent development: a long term follow up of 411 London males. In *Criminology: Personality, Behaviour, Life History* (eds H. J. Kerner & G. Kaiser). Heidelberg: Springer Verlag.

FAULK, M. (1988) *Basic Forensic Psychiatry*. Oxford: Blackwell Scientific.

FELDMANN, T. B., JOHN, P. W. & BELL, R. A. (1990) Cofactors in the commission of violent crimes. *American Journal of Psychotherapy*, **44**, 172–179.

FOTTRELL, E. (1980) A study of violent behaviour among patients in psychiatric hospitals. *British Journal of Psychiatry*, **136**, 216–221.

——, Bewley, T. & Squizzinoni, M. (1978) A study of aggressive and violent behaviour among a group of psychiatric in-patients. *Medicine, Sicence and the Law*, **18**, 66–69.

GUNN, J. (1982) Defining the terms.In *Dangerousness: Psychiatric Assessment and Management* (eds J. R. Hamilton & H. Freeman). pp 7–11. London: Gaskell.

—— (1991) Human violence: a biological perspective. *Criminal Behaviour and Mental Health*, **1**, 34–54.

HAFNER, H. & BOKER, W. (1973) Mentally disordered violent offenders. *Social Psychiatry*, **8**, 220–229.

HEALTH AND SAFETY ADVISORY COMMITTEE (1987) *Violence to Staff*. DHSS Advisory Committee on Violence to Staff Report. London: HMSO.

HEILBRUN, A. B., Jr. (1990) The measurement of criminal dangerousness as a personality constraint: further validation of a research index. *Journal of Personality Assessment*, **54**, 141–148.

HILL, G. (1985) Predicting recidivism using institutional measures. In *Prediction in Criminology* (eds D. P. Farrington & R. Tarling). Chichester: Wiley.

HODGKINSON, P. E., McIVOR, L. & PHILIPS, M. (1985) Patient assaults on staff in a psychiatric hospital: a two year retrospective study. *Medicine, Science and the Law*, **25**, 288–294.

HOME OFFICE AND DEPARTMENT OF HEALTH AND SOCIAL SECURITY (1975) *Report of the Committee on Mentally Abnormal Offenders* (Butler report, Cmnd 6244). London: HMSO.

IONNO, G. A. (1983) A prospective sutdy of assaultative behaviour in female psychiatric patients. In *Assaults within Psychiatric Hospitals* (eds J. R. Lion & W. H. Reid). New York: Grune & Stratton.

MacCULLOCH, M. J. & BAILEY, J. (1993) Issues in the management and rehabilitation of patients in maximum secure hospitals. *Journal of Forensic Psychiatry*, **4**, 25–44.

MADDEN, D. J., LION, J. R. & PENNA, M. W. (1976) Assaults on psychiatrists by patients. *American Journal of Psychiatry*, **133**, 422–425.

MANN, C. R. (1993) *Unequal Justice. A Question of Color*. USA: Indiana University Press.

MENZIES, R. J., WEBSTER, C. D. & SEPEJAK, D. S. (1985) The division of dangerousness: evaluating the accuracy of psychometric predictions of violence among forensic patients. *Law and Human Behaviour*, **9**, 35–56.

MONAHAN, J. (1988) Risk assessment of violence among the mentally disordered: generating useful knowledge. *International Journal of Law and Psychiatry*, **11**, 249–257.

OWENS, W. A. & SCHOENFELDT, L. F. (1979) Towards a classification of persons. *Journal of Applied Psychology*, **64**, 569–607.

PICKERSGILL, A. (1990) Balancing the private and public interests. In *Risk Taking in Mental Disorder* (ed. D. Carson). pp 23–27. England: SLE Publications.

QUINSEY, V. L., WARNEHEAD, A., PREUSSE, M. G., *et al* (1975) Released Oak Ridge patients: a follow up of review board discharges. *British Journal of Criminology*, **15**, 264–270.

Report on the Review of Procedures for the Discharge and Supervision of Psychiatric Patients Subject to Special Restrictions (1973) (Aarvold report). London: HMSO.

REVIEW OF HEALTH AND SOCIAL SERVICES FOR MENTALLY DISORDERED OFFENDERS AND OTHERS REQUIRING SIMILAR SERVICES (1992) *Final Summary Report*, cmnd 2088. London: HMSO.

RUBEN, I., WOLKAN, G. & YAMAMOTO, J. (1980) Physical attacks on psychiatric residents by patients. *Journal of Nervous and Mental Disease*, **168**, 243–345.

SCOTT, P. D. (1977) Assessing dangerousness in criminals. *British Journal of Psychiatry*, **131**, 127–142.

SNOWDEN, P. (1993) Taking risks (editorial). *Journal of Forensic Psychiatry*, **4**, 198–200.

STEADMAN, H. J. & COCOZZA, J. J. (1975) We can't predict who is dangerous. Psychology Today, 8, 32–35.

—— & —— (1983) The criminally insane patient: Who gets out? *Social Psychiatry*, **8**, 230–235.

TARDIFF, K. (1983) A survey of assaults by chronic patients ion a state mental system. In *Assaults Within Psychiatric Facilities* (eds J. R. Lyon & W. H. Reid). New York: Grune & Stratton.

TAYLOR, P. J. & GUNN, J. (1984) Violence and psychosis II – effect of psychiatric diagnosis on conviction and sentencing of offenders. *British Medical Journal*, **289**, 9–12.

WERNER, P. D. & PERRENCE, R. (1984) *Psychiatrists' judgement of dangerousness in patients on an acute care unit*. Rome: Yesavage, Kelleth & Seeman.

3   Interviewing the aggressive client

JEREMY COID

The purpose of this chapter is to enhance a professional's skills to cope with a potentially violent individual during an interview. This is just one facet of the management of a violent person. The chapter does not set out to introduce the reader to 'breakaway techniques' or detailed de-escalation strategies, which are discussed in Chapter 4, nor to discuss details of long-term management and medical treatment (dealt with in Chapter 5). Instead, the intention is to outline the basic principles, on the assumption that the reader will at some time have to carry out an interview with an aggressive person, or else will suddenly be faced with aggression during the course of an interview. In some cases it may be wiser not to carry out the interview at all. This chapter gives some indication of how to recognise when that is the case.

The first part of the chapter examines the importance of recognising and understanding our attitudes towards aggressive patients, evaluating the settings and resources necessary for the interview to take place, and the question of personal skills. This is essentially an examination of the basic principles when approaching the interview. The second part of the chapter presents a structured approach to the interview itself. This is derived from experience of working in settings where interviews with aggressive clients are frequent, and will not necessarily be appropriate to all situations and individuals. This model should generalise to a situation where aggression arises unexpectedly.

Management

Before discussing the process of interviewing, it is important to remember that the interview itself cannot be considered in isolation

27

from the overall management of an aggressive person. Interviewers may not be at a stage where they have overall responsibility for the person. Nevertheless, the interviewer does not merely require skills to cope with aggressive people, but must also be able to understand why they are behaving aggressively in the first place by analysing the problem, and assessing what facilities and resources are needed to cope and whether any changes in organisation are needed in the setting where the interview is taking place (Owens & Ashcroft, 1985; Breakwell, 1989). Other colleagues and professionals from different disciplines may have to be consulted to facilitate a successful plan of action over the long term.

Aggressive clients are usually complex, with a multitude of problems besides threatening behaviour and poor anger control (Roth, 1987). If professionals are confronted regularly with these individuals it is important to look carefully at their own management structure and position in the organisation. Have they received adequate training? Are adequate facilities provided to cope with difficult clients? Do they receive the supervision and personal support that is necessary in dealing with these difficult people? If the professional is part of a team, is that team sufficiently organised and oriented towards putting an effective plan into operation, or is the interviewer left to cope with a difficult client alone and without subsequent direction?

This chapter should help with difficult interviews in the short term, but if the answer to any of the above questions is in the negative, then it is reasonable for the professional to question whether he or she should be interviewing such individuals at all. Unless members of staff are clear about the direction in which they are going, and about the overall management policy for this group, their work will become increasingly stressful and demoralising, and it will be difficult and unsafe for them to work with this group of people.

Case example 3.1

A highly disturbed male, manic patient was admitted on a compulsory order of the Mental Health Act to a locked ward in a mental hospital. He had begun to show some improvement with medication, and three student nurses, who had recently started working on their first placement, were detailed to escort the patient in the grounds for some exercise. The patient encountered a female patient near the sports field and began to abuse her verbally with a stream of obscenities. When reprimanded by one of the nurses, the patient immediately punched him in the face, knocking him to the ground. The other two grappled with the patient and wrestled him to the ground. The first nurse then kicked the patient. On return to the ward the patient did not complain, and the nurses did not report the incident. However, it had been witnessed by a member of the public who did report it, and the nurse was suspended.

This incident makes the point that aggression between clients and professionals is not necessarily always one way, but is not presented for that reason. At the next multidisciplinary team meeting, some of the nursing staff roundly condemned their colleague's behaviour. However, it posed two important questions besides the professional qualities of the nurse concerned. First, what training had the three student nurses received in dealing with violent patients? Second, had it been a wise management decision to entrust unsupervised escorting duties of a disturbed patient to the three most inexperienced members of the clinical team? The role of the organisation in providing training is examined further in Chapter 6.

Preconceived attitudes

It is important to recognise that preformed and prejudged attitudes towards aggressive clients may make the situation worse and the interview more difficult. It is often forgotten that many aggressive clients are actually frightened themselves, and that their aggression can then stem from overwhelming feelings of passivity and helplessness, with imagined fears of the destruction of their own self-esteem and sometimes their own physical selves. If staff respond by an increasingly authoritarian stance or by counteraggression, this may increase the person's feelings of helplessness and increase the risk of consequent aggression. In some circumstances it may be necessary to use sufficient force to overwhelm a dangerous client in a crisis. Where this is not the case, and particularly when embarking on an interview designed to reduce a client's aggression, it is important to be aware of negative attitudes.

Negative attitudes may be shared by a staff team as a whole or be held by the individual who has to carry out the interview. Conflicts between team members and shared fantasies about a client's dangerousness can undermine the professional's ability to cope in an objective manner. Staff may have prejudices based on socio-economic, racial, ethnic, or educational aspects of the client, leading to fantasies or stereotyped expectations of behaviour. Staff can also develop attitudes or feelings based on a single piece of history or behaviour before they have even seen the client. If this leads them to expect the worse, then they may start to respond with increasing anxiety and anger, the subsequent response on meeting the client may be punitive, repressive, or neglecting, and this may actually provoke violence (Dubin, 1989).

Case example 3.2

A patient suffering from schizophrenia was readmitted after a further relapse of his illness on an emergency hospital order signed by his general practitioner and a social worker. On his first admission he had assaulted a nurse and had once served a term of imprisonment for a serious attack on a member of his family. A psychiatric report contained in his case notes stated that should there be further violence, a second opinion should be sought with a view to transfer to a maximum-security hospital. Uncertain of the circumstances of the admission, additional nursing staff were sent to the receiving ward, where there was considerable apprehension about his arrival. Upon his arrival he was told that his belongings would be searched for weapons and that no aggression would be tolerated. He became angry and abusive and was immediately restrained and placed in seclusion room where he remained for several days, receiving large doses of tranquillising medication. He was later transferred in a drowsy state to a secure unit where medication was reduced and the patient remained well. He made steady progress and remained a 'model patient'.

It is important to evaluate what is known about the client objectively and not attribute a 'larger than life' reputation for dangerousness when it is unwarranted. On the other hand it is foolish to minimise obvious risks from information available and not take sensible precautions when they are required.

A colleague who has interviewed a client before and talks disparagingly about another professional's anxiety may not only act in an insensitive manner, but may well never have touched on the person's true underlying problem and aggression. Be wary of colleagues who proudly assert that they have a 'good' or 'special' relationship with a potentially dangerous client. They may be bolstering their own self-esteem and colluding with the more negative features of a client's psychopathology. Wider aspects of dangerousness are discussed in Chapter 2.

Inexperienced staff should not assume that there is always a right way of dealing with an aggressive client. More experienced colleagues may well have better skills from practice, but it is not a hard-and-fast rule that they will always be successful with every difficult encounter. If an interviewer gets into difficulties there may well be no 'right' way of behaving, just an ability to keep thinking until the next step is found, sometimes intuitively. Similarly, inexperienced interviewers should not feel that anxiety and fear are inappropriate reactions when confronted by these individuals, or that such feelings have to be suppressed at all costs. It is obvious that an interview cannot be conducted in a state of panic, but once experience is gained the feeling of anxiety in the presence of a difficult client can be monitored carefully, and these feelings can tell us what is going on and how the interview is progressing.

Assessing resources

If the reader has never considered what he/she would do if confronted with a potentially violent client then it is perhaps time to do so. By rehearsing in your mind how to deal with aggression you may find it easier to deal with the real thing.

The first rule when approaching such an encounter is that no interview can be successful unless the interviewer feels confident. It is therefore important to consider what resources are available to feel confident. Does the interviewer have sufficient personal experience and training to conduct such an interview? Has he/she been taught how to calm agitated clients, watched others doing it, or had the opportunity to sit in while a more experienced colleague interviews a difficult client? The more personal experience the interviewer has, the easier it will be to cope if aggression occurs unexpectedly. In addition, the more likely a professional is to meet aggressive individuals in their everyday working life then the more they will need this experience.

Have readers ever looked at their office, ward, or general environment in which they work and considered what they could do if threatened or attacked? Could they escape if necessary? Could the alarm be raised if a client got out of control? Would colleagues be aware of their whereabouts? Is the interview being conducted in a room near to colleagues, in case help is needed, and are interviews always carried out before colleagues have gone home for the evening? Do colleagues have contingency plans that would be put into operation in the event of a violent incident? If the answer to any of these is 'no', then professional confidence will inevitably be reduced and if they have to interview the client then their effectiveness in controlling the situation may well be reduced, with consequent risks to their safety.

In a situation where a home visit is contemplated, the professional has least control over the environment and may be at considerably more risk than in a hospital or institution. It is in the client's home where the professional is at greatest disadvantage. The client has more control over the environment, and other persons may be present. It may be a completely unknown environment and if the individual's mental state is also unknown there is a need for much greater caution. Professionals should decide whether it is really safe, whether factors in the purpose of the visit may actually be provocative in themselves, whether they should be accompanied, and even whether the visit is necessary. If there may be difficulties, the professional should be aware of exits in the vicinity. Davies (1989) makes the important recommendation that colleagues should always be aware of when and where the professional visited.

Office layout and design

It is well worth paying careful attention to the details of the room in which the interview takes place. The client needs to feel secure and relaxed, as does the interviewer, who has to remain in control and not allow a potentially violent client to dominate the space. The room should be the right size: not so large that the client can readily get up and pace around; on the other hand, it can be a highly uncomfortable experience to interview a paranoid or threatening client in close proximity within a cramped office. The fixtures and decoration should not be oppressive and should be conducive to relaxation. Potential weapons and missiles such as ornaments or a heavy ashtray should be removed. Remember, any freshly delivered hot cup of coffee from the waiting-room vending machine should be drunk, with polite encouragement, before the interview commences.

Pay careful attention to the position of the chairs. It is inadvisable to sit face to face with an aggressive client in a confronting or 'eyeball to eyeball' position. Sit roughly at 45° or place the chairs where patient and interviewer can look at and away from each other comfortably, without appearing evasive, shifty, or confrontational. Some interviewers prefer a desk. This can be placed as a 'barrier' between client and interviewer and may give a feeling of relief and protection, but this will also reduce the ability to make emotional contact and will reduce the amount of control over what is happening on the other side. Placing the patient beside the desk allows the interview to be conducted at 45°, with more contact, but lends a degree of formality to the procedure (Fig. 3.1).

Choice of chairs is also highly important. It is preferable for the interviewer to have a slightly higher and harder chair than the client, preferably without sides so that if it is necessary to get out of one's seat quickly, it is easier to move sideways and does not appear as if the interviewer is coming at the client. Offer the client a softer,

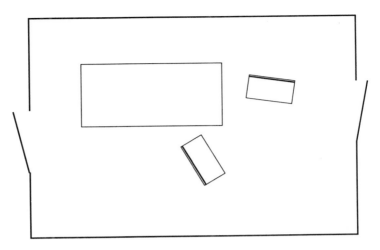

Fig. 3.1   An ideal office layout for interviewing potentially aggressive people

more comfortable, lower chair. If the reader tries this out by changing places it becomes clear how much more difficult it is to intimidate another person looking upwards from a soft base. It is therefore highly inadvisable to conduct an interview with the client standing, a position from which it is easier to escalate into violence. Always encourage the client to sit or return to a seated position during the interview. It may be advisable to terminate the interview if the patient will not remain seated. One further point to remember is that many paranoid and agitated people feel more comfortable with a wall behind them.

Both interviewer and client should be able to get to the door without blocking one another. This will allow the interviewer to escape if it becomes necessary and clients to storm out in anger if they feel they have to, without having to push the interviewer out of the way. In a working environment where aggressive clients or 'unknown quantities' are frequently encountered, it is helpful to have an office with two doors at opposite corners. At least one should have an unbreakable window so that colleagues can check on one's safety without intruding or disrupting the interview. The door should not have a lock which can be operated from the inside without a key and prevent rescue. The key itself should never be left in the lock. The door should also be outward opening to prevent barricading from within by an angry client holding the interviewer hostage.

It may be advisable to have a 'panic' button placed in a reachable position for the interviewer and connected to a central point where colleagues can be alerted if difficulties occur. These are rarely used in most hospitals or other care establishments, but they offer the staff the reassurance that help could be summoned if it became necessary. The use of electronic alarms is discussed further in Chapter 6.

Having colleagues present

When an interview cannot be avoided and if there is a real risk of assault from the client, then it would be foolish not to have others present. In these circumstances it is essential to have skilled and overwhelming force available to control the client without injury. In less pressing situations it is still reasonable for professionals to set themselves a rule that they do not interview clients alone when they do not feel comfortable. A successful outcome can only be achieved if the interviewer feels confident.

Choose carefully when having a colleague or colleagues present. A large male colleague sitting quietly in the room may make the interviewer feel more secure but sometimes can act as a focus for a client's aggression. Some male clients can be handled without difficulty by a confident female adopting a challenging but motherly manner in a situation where a male would elicit frank hostility. On the other hand, this may be a provocative combination for a person with a history of paranoid beliefs about women or a history of sexual assaults on women. At the same time, if there is to be more than one member of staff present it is important to establish beforehand who is in charge of the interview and whether there will be any interaction between staff, so as not to confuse the client.

Case example 3.3

A male psychiatrist was called to see a disturbed prisoner in the segregation unit. He had been moved from another prison to a special unit for psychiatric observation of inmates thought to have mental health problems. He was currently serving a seven-year sentence for a brutal sexual assault on a woman and had a history of similar offences. He had been totally unable to conform and demonstrate acceptable behaviour in the other prison, where he had spent most of his time in solitary confinement in the segregation unit. He only lasted a matter of hours in the assessment unit and was too disturbed and threatening to interview when first seen in his cell, the doctor having to be flanked in the doorway by four prison officers. He voluntarily accepted tranquillising medication and requested next day to have a further interview. He appeared calm and was seen alone. He informed the doctor that he could not tolerate the presence of female staff in the assessment unit and went on to inform him coldly that he would assault him, inflicting as much damage as possible before officers could intervene, if he did not receive the doctor's word that transfer back the original prison could be arranged.

This is an extreme and unusual case but demonstrates that exceptionally dangerous psychopaths and those with nothing to lose from their behaviour are capable of inflicting considerable injury if it suits their purpose. It had been a mistake to interview this particular individual without staff present in the room, in view of what was already known about him. In the event, the interview had taken place with the prison officers a relatively short distance away in the corridor, and the doctor had a radio-controlled alarm attached to his belt. In the face of the prisoner's threats the doctor wisely conceded to the demand and terminated the interview quickly.

One additional advantage in having colleagues present is the prevention of the client losing contact with reality and incorporating the interviewer into bizarre beliefs. Some clients have a tenuous hold on reality as a result of acute psychosis or stress in combination with an unstable personality. Their ideas may be influenced by early traumatic experiences. Delusions or hallucinations may establish a bizarre and frightening psychotic transference onto the interviewer, who may be perceived quite differently or as someone else. Having a colleague present can give some relief to both client and interviewer from this situation, especially if it is known to have manifested on a previous occasion.

Client–professional interactions

Having assessed the resources available, it is helpful to briefly consider what is happening during an interview. It is essential when carrying out the procedure with an aggressive person that the interviewer maintains a sense of purpose and is not diverted from this by the patient. There are established patterns in which professionals learn to behave towards their clients during their training, and in the behaviour that is expected in return.

One observer believes that self-preservation takes place by what he calls a series of 'quasi-theatrical' performances, in which there is a collusion between those who are interacting. Argyle (1975) has described 'rules' which regulate the coordination and sequence of events. It is only by adhering to these rules that the special professional–client relationship can continue. This will allow the situation where, for example, doctors and nurses can touch and examine intimate parts of patients' bodies and where particularly sensitive questions can be asked within an interview. If the rules are broken, particularly where violence towards the professional is threatened, then the sequence of normal events is dislocated and the professional may no longer be able to continue. It is therefore important to be aware of and to stick to these 'rules'.

Body language

There is an exchange of messages in all social interactions, many of which are conveyed and registered at an unconscious level. Non-verbal communication of emotions is largely innate, partly because of the direct effect of physiological states and because of the development of social signals. Among animals, the adaptive purpose of non-verbal communication is to keep other members of the social group continuously informed about their inner states, but it also displays the level of dominance of one animal over another. Attitude towards others is demonstrated by the nature of the gaze, the degree of proximity, and posture. Dominance in relation to higher or lower social status can be partly communicated by the relative pattern of bodily relaxation and asymmetrical body posture, for example where one person has one hand in a pocket and is casually reclining in contrast to the other person.

During the interview with an aggressive individual it there is a subtle competition of signals which negotiate at the non-verbal level the precise relationship between the two persons, with many of the client's signals effectively seeking to establish dominance over the interviewer. Some awareness of body language is important in gauging the interview's progress. For example, increasing dominance by the patient may be accompanied by increasing tension and immobility in the interviewer, with submissive head lowered and rounded shoulders in marked contrast to the increasing upper limb movements and prolonged gazing of the patient. On the other hand, progressive relaxation in the posture of both may indicate progress towards a satisfactory outcome.

During the interview it is important to be aware of eye-to-eye gaze, and this has been partly addressed already in the position of chairs. Prolonged staring may be perceived as a challenge by an aggressive client, yet avoidance of eye-to-eye contact may be perceived as evasiveness or shiftiness. It is best to proceed somewhere in between, with regular but not prolonged glances at the client, increasing the length and intensity of the gaze when making important points or expressing care and concern. A posture with head lowered and rounded shoulders signals submission and can be demonstrated in response to angry outbursts from the client. Alternating from the submissive position to a more upright and direct posture can allow the interviewer to 'ride' the fluctuating emotions of the client during the early stages.

Another important aspect of body language is that it will convey powerful messages about the interviewer's attitude – lack of concern is not only conveyed by what the interviewer says. This can lead to escalating disturbance if clients feel they are getting no response.

Apparent anger in the interviewer may also lead to relaxation. Empathy can be conveyed by leaning slightly towards clients to express concern when they show features indicating distress. Need for closeness will vary between clients. Paranoid individuals will find this particularly difficult to tolerate. On the other hand, intoxicated clients will sometimes tolerate a closeness which would be quite unacceptable under normal circumstances.

Inner perceptions

Interviewing aggressive clients can be a highly stressful experience even for the most experienced professional. These individuals can create a range of different emotions and feelings in the interviewer, all of which are normal reactions, and professionals should not feel embarrassed about them. It is important to be aware of these and monitor them, as they may convey a considerable amount of information about the client and will help guide the interview.

Anger

It is essential to recognise anger and deal with this, avoiding provocation and responding to insults. On some occasions it may be acceptable to express anger towards a client in a constructive manner – for example, "perhaps people behave like that towards you because you frighten them and they get angry towards you in return" – or as a means to set limits on unacceptable behaviour – "I can't help you if you are going to keep shouting". It may be more appropriate to divert clients on to topics which make them less angry during the difficult parts of the interview and return to more sensitive issues when their anger is under control.

Fear

An interviewer should not approach an aggressive individual with the attitude that he/she must never show fear and that it is essential to remain entirely calm and relaxed at all times. If it can be achieved this is fine, but it is usually not possible. Struggling with attempts to contain such emotions may give a misleading impression to the client. Fear of the aggressive person is a natural response which can only be reduced by confidence in the interview setting and situation, one's own personal abilities, and increased knowledge and understanding of the client. Increasing experience of successful interviews with aggressive people and the careful use of resources, such as having others present, can help reduce feelings of fear. However, one should not aim to eliminate all feelings of anxiety, as they can help to measure how the interview is progressing. A sudden, unexpected feeling of fear does not necessarily indicate a fault in the interviewer's technique or a serious failure of courage. It may be an important sign or even the only warning sign of impending violence.

Case example 3.4

A junior doctor was interviewing a patient with paranoid schizophrenia who had referred himself to a psychiatric emergency clinic. She had elicited his main complaints, his personal history, and many of the symptoms of his psychotic illness, but felt that he was not revealing all his hallucinatory and delusional experiences. He asked her an occasional question about herself but otherwise was not particularly inappropriate or intrusive in his manner. As the interview progressed she became increasingly uncomfortable for no reason she could identify. Eventually she became increasingly fearful of the patient. Intuitively, she decided to stop the interview and leave the room, making a polite excuse. As she walked along the corridor from the interviewing room towards the nurses at the reception desk the patient followed her, came up quickly from behind, and punched her in the face, knocking her to the ground.

The doctor's intuition was not the result of what the patient said, but the unconscious registering of a series of non-verbal messages from the patient's body language and subtle changes in his manner and mood. These betrayed his growing hostility and violent intentions, which were the result of his paranoid ideas, now incorporating the doctor. Leaving the interview room was clearly the only course of action in the face of this growing feeling of fear. If an interviewer suspects that a client is deliberating on whether to carry out an assault there is no alternative.

Confusion

With a particularly difficult client, when the interviewer appears to be getting nowhere, or with a client who talks about distasteful, emotionally charged or violent material for a prolonged period, the interviewer may gradually feel overcome with a sensation of mental numbness or confusion. It is as if the client has overloaded the interviewer so that he/she can no longer think clearly. In these circumstances, it is important to observe a fixed time for the interview or to terminate at this point, if only for a break if the interviewer feels able to change the direction. Having a colleague present the next time may be helpful, and it is advisable to discuss the management of such clients with a supervisor or colleague later to check that work is progressing in the right direction.

Fatigue

Interviews with aggressive clients are among the most tiring and emotionally draining of experiences, requiring a high level of concentration which must be maintained for longer than usual. It is undesirable to have a large caseload of such individuals or that the responsibility for them should always fall upon one member of the team. If there can be a coffee break then the time to take it is after seeing one of these clients.

The interview

This chapter has so far conveyed some understanding of the effects that aggressive individuals can have on professionals and some of the precautions that need to be taken. However, many readers will not consider it their professional role to set out even to conduct a formal interview with such a client. In some working environments this may be difficult to avoid however. Because of the nature of the caring professions, people who present in an aggressive manner may be perceived as asking for help or may even have been referred for treatment of their aggression. The nature of the professional's role may then be to assess the client and carry out a plan of management. It is therefore important that interviewers maintain their professional role throughout, but are aware of the limitations of what can actually be offered. For example, hospitals are not providers of accommodation or money, and social workers do not provide medication. An aggressive client may be exerting considerable pressure to get the professional to concede to demands and yet may have officially presented for the purpose of obtaining the professional's help.

The rest of the chapter suggests a model for approaching the interview itself. This covers broader issues than the medical management of patients (discussed in Chapter 5), and complements the strategies discussed in Chapter 4.

The model presented in this chapter can be divided into three stages:

   (a) Stage I. Assessment and calming the client
      (i)   pre-interview assessment
      (ii)   personal introduction
      (iii) calming the client
      (iv) eliciting main problems
   (b) Stage II. History taking and counselling
      (i)   re-evaluation of direction and purpose of interview
      (ii)   further clarification of main issues
      (iii) working through anger
   (c) Stage III. Formulation and termination
      (i)   formulate main problems for client
      (ii)   agree on possible solutions
      (iii) termination

In presenting this model there are two necessary caveats. First, the model is intended to be flexible and readily modified to fit in with the professional model that the reader already applies as a result of professional training – for example social case work for a social worker, nursing process for nursing staff, clinical history taking for doctors. Second, it should not be thought of as a rigid model that applies to every individual or situation. For example, with clients known to be dangerous or in a highly disturbed state, it may be inadvisable even to attempt to proceed to the second stage. An interview incorporating stage I and a shortened stage III may be all that is possible. For readers who do not see their professional role as involving regular interviews with aggressive clients, the various principles described below, rather than the three-stage framework itself, are likely to be of greater interest.

Stage I. Assessment and calming the client

Before seeing any client who is known to be aggressive, it is essential to obtain as much objective information as possible from records and other sources. For example, a telephone call to another professional may explain why the person is creating a disturbance in the waiting-room. This gives interviewers time to assess their resources and decide on a strategy to deal with the client. It is important to be aware of how clients' attitudes may have been influenced by what happened upon their arrival, before the interview began. Have they been waiting long? Have other colleagues (receptionists etc.) been treating them politely? This may have to be dealt with and discussed at some stage of the interview.

Behaviour and demeanour should be observed before and during the personal introduction. For example, clients may have made a threat to a colleague or banged their fists on the waiting-room wall. They may be intoxicated, and if so it is sometimes necessary to ask these clients to return when sober. They may be too volatile and aroused for an interview to be conducted in safety.

Personal introduction is usually the first interaction and can profoundly influence the rest of the interview. This should be polite and formal if it is for the first time. It tells clients who you are and what your role is in seeing them – for example, "Hello, I'm Doctor XY, I was asked by the staff to come and see you because you appeared to be distressed. What can I do to help you?" Sometimes clients may need to be told at an early stage that violent behaviour cannot be tolerated if they are to be helped.

Some individuals may be so disturbed they are unable to reply at first to the interviewer's questions and may have to be calmed and reassured before a formal interview can begin. Once the request is made for clients to say what is troubling them, their response is rather like the opening gambit of a chess game. A statement of distress or anger, even if they cannot explain the reason for their feelings, indicates a direction for further explanation. An immediate demand, such as drugs or a certain course of action from the interviewer, such as "I want you to telephone my wife and tell her I'm not mad!", warrants caution before proceeding further. It may be necessary to state the 'rules', for example, "I'm not a doctor, I can't prescribe drugs", or "Perhaps I need to know a bit more about you and your problems before I can decide to . . .".

When clients are angry and aroused they should be encouraged to sit and to remain seated if they wish to stand. Encourage them to try to relax and talk about their problems. It may be necessary to offer medication and even to ask the client to have a 'walk around' outside the interviewing room (not in front of the interviewer) to get control of their emotions if this is proving difficult. Do not interview with other persons present who are also angry or aroused, as they may escalate the client's anger further. It is usually best to see clients alone unless there is a caring relative or friend who is known to have a calming influence, or in the case of the client who is afraid of the interviewer.

Try to find out how the client felt about coming. Doubts and fears about the interview itself and its outcome may be allayed at the outset, although no promises should be made before more information is obtained. Once the person can be persuaded to explain what is making him/her angry, display empathy by expressing concern, paraphrasing if necessary what the person has said, and reflecting on feelings, for example, "Yes, I can see that it made you very angry". Finally, try to discover what the aggression is directed towards: is it a specific person who has enraged the client or is the client in a general state of anger which could be directed at anyone, including the interviewer?

Stage II. History taking and counselling

If the individual's problems or general demeanour are beyond the interviewer's resources, then the interview should be terminated. At this stage the interviewer should be clear about the direction in which the interview will be going and its purpose. Most professionals will have training in eliciting the necessary information for their professional role, and at this stage the interviewer requires as much information as possible (or is practical in the circumstances) to move to the final stage. It may be necessary to go over the individual's presenting complaints, what brought them to the interview, and their current social situation (housing, relationships, employment, etc.). The professional is attempting to understand the nature of the person's aggressive behaviour and its origins. The personal and family history may include violence and abuse from parental figures and family members, or the witnessing of violence between them. If it is possible to obtain information on the person's upbringing and longitudinal development, including factors relating to aggression and impulse control, this will help in formulating the problems and planning a course of action at the next stage.

During this second stage, the interviewer may decide to counsel the person and help with the immediate problem of angry feelings. The aim is gradually to reduce the level of anger and arousal by getting clients to express their feelings and frustrations in a controlled manner. This can be time-consuming and stressful. Some clients will visibly relax and settle as they begin to talk about their problems. Others become more volatile and angry when sensitive issues are touched upon. The interviewer may have to move away from these issues and then return to them according to the client's mood. Many clients are genuinely afraid and confused by the feelings and emotions themselves. They may fear that they are 'going mad' or 'cracking up', and may be reassured to learn that what they are experiencing are normal, if somewhat extreme, emotions expressed by everyone in stressful situations. For some clients the interviewer will act like a teacher, explaining to them what they are actually experiencing and the links between these emotions and the life events they have experienced. It is often surprising for inexperienced professionals to discover that these links, which appear to be obvious to the observer, are in fact totally absent from the cognitions of many individuals. This is typically seen in personality-disordered clients or those from severely deprived backgrounds, particularly when they are under stress.

Maintaining control

Aggressive individuals often try to change the 'rules' of the relationship between professional and client . Much of the verbal expression and body language is effective in dominating the space around them and the persons within it. However, if the interviewer cannot maintain control of the situation, the goals of the second and third stages of the interview cannot be met. The interviewer must maintain the boundaries between what is acceptable and what is not acceptable, and these must be reaffirmed in various ways without provocative confrontation. As has already been explained, this can be done by telling clients that violence cannot be tolerated or that the interview cannot continue if they keep shouting. It may also be done by inference, for example by reassuring them that their legal rights will not be taken away and that they cannot therefore be compulsorily detained because they are not mentally ill and are therefore responsible for all their actions. By inference, violence would therefore be dealt with by the law, from which they will not have an excuse on the grounds of mental illness.

It is essential that both parties stick within the 'rules' of the professional–client relationship. It should also be a rule that once the interviewer begins to lose control, or feels increasingly dominated by the client, that the interview is terminated. A situation should not be reached from which there may be no returning. Colleagues who have got into difficulties with their clients have described some of the following warning signs.

(i) Frozen fearfulness

This is a progressive anxiety and fearfulness in the interviewer, with loss of awareness and control over what is happening. It is important to remain flexible in one's thinking throughout the interview and to be able to keep thinking if things seem to be going wrong. It is best to leave the interview well before clarity of thought is lost. (See also Chapter 4.)

(ii) Dehumanisation

It is easier to assault someone who does not have normal, likable human qualities. Watch out for indications that the client is dehumanising the interviewer, such as: "Social workers are all scum, they took my children away"; "Call yourself a doctor? You're trash"; "People who treat me like that deserve everything they get". It may help to personalise oneself, sometimes giving certain details about oneself, rather than just the detail of a characterless professional. But if the situation is escalating, terminate the interview.

(iii) Failure to follow the client's train of thought

With a very disturbed or psychotic person this may be difficult anyway, but when it becomes increasingly frequent or is a deteriorating feature it may indicate that the person is rapidly losing contact with reality or may be deliberately withholding pieces of information and playing with the interviewer.

(iv) Point of no return

A point can be reached in the interview where there is no possibility of returning to the normal rules of a professional–client relationship. It may become manifest with increasingly suggestive speech content, sexual innuendoes, increasing physical proximity, and especially if the person physically touches the interviewer in an inappropriate manner. This is the point to terminate.

Stage III. Formulation and termination

If the interviewer has helped to decrease the client's level of arousal and has collected sufficient information, then a formulation can be made of the person's main problems. It is important to give an explanation of your professional opinion in words the person can understand. List the problems and potential solutions or alternative courses of action. This may not be easy with clients who have set their minds on something else, who may not like the options, or who try to shift the interview back a phase. Be firm. Point out the limitations of what can be offered and resist going back over the same ground. It may be necessary to set in motion a particular plan of action, such as arranging urgent hospital admission, or prescribing medication – which may make termination easier. If clients are reluctant to leave because they have not achieved what they wanted, it is still important to terminate firmly and not to return to the second stage. Make it clear what further follow-up, if any, there will be. Explain politely but firmly that any new issues that the client suddenly raises will have to be looked at next time.

Case example 3.5

A young man had recently been released from prison, having served a sentence for assault. He had a long history of violence, including two serious assaults on nurses during previous admissions. His consultant had diagnosed him as a psychopath and banned him from the ward on the grounds that psychiatry had nothing further to offer him. His imminent reappearance at the hospital emergency clinic was announced by a female patient who had briefly accommodated him in her flat and whom he had subsequently tried to strangle during sexual intercourse. She was now requesting admission herself to get away from him. He was 'interviewed' at the top of the hospital steps, outside the clinic, by a junior doctor and nurse and requested to return in the afternoon to see a more senior member of staff. Later that day he was seen by a more experienced psychiatrist accompanied by a male nurse and social worker. The interview was extremely frightening for all three staff. The patient threatened them with violence if admission could not be arranged or money provided. At one stage the patient appeared to lose contact with reality. Little could be understood, but he seemed to think he was back in prison and that one of the prisoners in the cell was making homosexual advances to him. He acted out a demonstration of how he would cut his throat and wrists, showing multiple scars from previous self-mutilating episodes. He then talked of persecutory voices and the delusional belief that he was a pop star. The psychiatrist barely maintained control of the interview but elicited sufficient information to decide that the man was psychotic, and probably suffering from schizophrenia. He recommended medication in a long-acting injection which, to his surprise and relief, the patient readily accepted. The social worker obtained a place for him in a hostel for the homeless and the patient was offered a follow-up appointment a week later. Over the next six weeks the patient showed a marked improvement in his attitude and demeanour. He was finally referred to another consultant in the forensic psychiatry department, by which time his mental state was much better.

This case illustrates many of the features already discussed in the chapter. To some extent the patient's reputation for dangerous behaviour was justified by previous behaviour. It was appropriate to interview him with more than one person present and the interview might have ended disastrously if the doctor had seen him alone. It should be remembered that when one department or agency refuses to accept responsibility for a difficult client, that person does not necessarily go away. Another department or agency may have to take up the responsibility instead. In this case, a shortened version of stage II of the interview was employed, as the man was too volatile to attempt to calm by verbal means. The best that could be done was to offer medication. Issues of homelessness and destitution were as important in the man's presentation as eliciting the symptoms of his psychotic illness which had been missed by other professionals. However, by tolerating this difficult interview the simple intervention of starting medication and finding accommodation had been so successful that by the time the forensic psychiatrist took over the man's long-term management he stated that he could not see what "all the fuss" had been about.

Conclusions

With experience and confidence it is possible to cope successfully with many aggressive individuals during an interview. Individuals who behave aggressively are often profoundly distressed and later grateful for the opportunity to have shared their problems with a caring professional who is able to make sense of the chaos of their emotions and experiences. However, this is a stressful experience for a professional and risks should not be taken. It should be a rule that no aggressive client is interviewed unless the professional feels confident about his/her own safety. Should control begin to slip away during the interview, then it should be terminated. The core principles of systematic de-escalation discussed in Chapter 4 will also help during such an interview.

One sobering aspect should always be accepted when working with these difficult people. The interviewer may have developed the necessary skills and confidence, and may have maintained control and coped with the client throughout the interview, but this still may not be enough.

Case example 3.6

A young woman of low IQ had done a considerable amount of damage to a hostel after a row with another resident, and was told by staff to find accommodation elsewhere. Two hours later she presented to a psychiatric hospital demanding admission. She alternated between threats to the interviewing doctor and towards herself. Admission was refused and no amount of counselling could calm her when she could not get what she wanted. She refused an emergency placement in another hostel for the homeless. Finally, she stormed out of the interview and lay down in the road outside the hospital. When the police arrived, she jumped to her feet, punched one, and ripped the other's uniform. When it was established by the officers that she was

Summary points

- Be aware of your own attitudes: preconceived views can affect the way you deal with a client and can make violence more likely.
- Consider your own training and experience, the support available and the safety of the surroundings. Does office furniture need to be rearranged to increase ease of escape? Would another room be more suitable, for example one closer to other staff, or with two exits? Are there potential weapons which need to be removed, such as heavy ashtrays or cups of hot coffee? Is it necessary to ask a colleague to join the interview? Do other staff know that a potentially dangerous interview is in progress?
- If making a home visit, consider the risks even more carefully. Make sure that a colleague knows your location and expected time of return. Do not interview a client alone if you do not feel comfortable.
- The interview should follow the stages assessment and calming of the client, history taking and counselling, and formulation and termination, but be flexible: if necessary abbreviate the interview, or modify its aims.
- Obtain as much information as possible beforehand. Telephone other professionals for information about the client before proceeding. Observe the person's behaviour before taking him/her into an interview room. Introduce yourself politely and state the reason for the interview, explaining your role.
- Be aware of your posture and degree of eye contact, and that of the person being interviewed, throughout. Do not ignore feelings of anxiety or fear: unexplained anxiety may be an indication of potential danger.
- If you seem to be losing control of the interview, terminate it.
- Assuming you are able to proceed with the interview satisfactorily, bring the interview to a clear conclusion. Explain your opinion in words which the person can understand. Resist going back over the same ground with an increasingly aroused person.
- Be realistic in your expectations of what you can achieve in an interview.

not an in-patient and not considered by the doctor to be mentally ill she was arrested and taken away, struggling and screaming. She was later charged with assault and criminal damage.

There should be a limit to the interviewer's expectations of what can be achieved. It is best to have simple goals for these difficult clients over the short term. The aggressive client will often present multiple problems to the interviewer that cannot all be dealt with. Sometimes this will include a personal challenge to the professional, including the question of what the professional role entails. It is perhaps not surprising that the doctor in the example above felt considerable guilt for not preventing the arrest of this woman, and subsequently debated with himself whether admission should have been arranged. By presenting at the hospital she had become a 'patient' and the doctor's 'role' was to help her. However, unless professionals have a realistic awareness of their personal limitations and those of the institution or organisation they work for, then attempts to help aggressive individuals will not be successful.

References

ARGYLE, M. (1975) *Bodily Communications*. London: Methuen.
BREAKWELL, G. (1989) *Facing Physical Violence*. London: British Psychological Society and Routledge.
DAVIES, W. (1989) The prevention of assault on professional helpers. In *Clinical Approaches to Violence* (eds K. Howells & C. R. Hollin). Chichester: Wiley.
DUBIN, W. R. (1989) The role of fantasies, countertransference, and psychological defences in patient violence. *Hospital and Community Psychiatry*, **40**, 1280–1283.
OWENS, R. G. & ASHCROFT, J. B. (1985) *Violence: A Guide for the Caring Professions*. London: Croom Helm.
ROTH, L. H. (1987) *Clinical Treatment of the Violent Person*. New York: Guilford Publications.

4 De-escalating aggressive behaviour

DAVID LEADBETTER and BRODIE PATERSON

Social workers, nursing, medical, paramedical and housing staff have been murdered by clients in the UK in recent years. These deaths have prompted a range of initiatives including government reports, conferences, publications, and research initiatives (e.g. Brown *et al*, 1986; Crane, 1986; Rowett, 1986; National Union of Public Employees, 1991; Leadbetter, 1993*c*). Despite this attention, understanding of the scale of the problem is restricted by continuing under-reporting of incidents (Wenk *et al*, 1972; Lion *et al*, 1981; Stark & Kidd, 1992), which is fuelled by a range of unhelpful beliefs and attitudes (Lanza, 1983; Crane, 1986; Leadbetter, 1993*c*).

Attitudes to violence

This chapter deals with strategies for de-escalation, and with physical breakaway techniques. The use of these techniques must be put in the context of organisational responses to violence, and of individual attitudes to assault. Staff may feel that, if they are involved in an assault, it indicates a lack of competence on their part. If these views are shared by management and by other staff, they tend to focus the search for the causes of and solutions to violent behaviour exclusively on the skills and competence of staff (Johnstone, 1988). Individual attitudes can feed into this, with beliefs which either promote confrontation – "I must win", "Violence must not go unpunished" – or avoidance – "I can't cope", "I need a man to help with this situation". These attitudes can help to define 'aggression management' as an exclusively male or female trait, rather than a professional skill. They can also be used to rationalise abusive staff behaviour, which in turn can produce a confrontational unit culture which engenders violence and results in further staff defensiveness.

These factors, which tend to individualise violence, ignore wider issues, such as the pathological roots of violent behaviour, power disparities between staff and clients, and the limited support and training available to many public sector workers. This chapter discusses the interpersonal skills and tactics involved in effective aggression management. It is important to remember that these techniques are only one of the responses required to deal with aggression. Contextual matters such as the legal and moral responsibilities of employing agencies and their managers are not dealt with here. Effective responses to all forms of abusive behaviour must involve the development of appropriate practices and a 'shared ethos' across agencies, units, teams and individuals within a framework of appropriate policies, adequate resources, effective management and staff support and training.

Effective de-escalation

The concept of de-escalation, sometimes also referred to as 'defusing' or 'talk down', is simple. It refers to a set of verbal and non-verbal responses which, if used selectively and appropriately, reduce the level of a person's hostility by reducing anger and the predisposition to assaultive behaviour (Turnbull *et al*, 1990).

There is no standard approach to the de-escalation of aggression. The absence of systematic research on the content and effectiveness of current approaches makes it difficult to draw conclusions about the nature of effective staff responses applicable across professional settings. Against this background of uncertainty, a range of models and training programmes have emerged, few of which have been systematically evaluated.

Competing methods of de-escalation result from the complexity of the issue and the lack of consensus around the factors and processes which give rise to violent behaviour. Although the existing theories do not readily lend themselves to synthesis (Siann, 1985), the concept of de-escalation implies the adoption of an ecological approach, which views a violent event as an interplay between the aggressor, the potential victim, and the circumstances in which the confrontation occurs (Steadman, 1982; Stevenson, 1991).

A useful and simple conceptual model is provided by Bailey (1977), who adopts a fire-fighting analogy. This suggests that a violent incident requires four distinct elements, and that the removal of any one element stops the violence:

(a) a *target* – this can be a staff member, fellow client or the aggressor him/herself
(b) a *weapon*, whether an object, a limb or fist, foot, etc.
(c) a *trigger*, or stimulus, which releases aggression
(d) a state of *arousal.*

The role of targets and weapons are clear. Some of the attitudes and beliefs discussed above may make staff reluctant to withdraw from threatening situations and thus remove the target. Similarly, risk denial may delay staff in recognising the range of objects within clinical and care settings which can be used as weapons. The concepts of triggers and arousal are of particular importance in understanding the process of de-escalation.

Triggers

Victims often fail to anticipate violent behaviour, despite overt signs of hostility. This may be because their own judgement is impaired by the emotions stirred by the situation, or because the triggers are not obvious at the time. Although the identification of triggers is often done in retrospect, knowledge of a client's behaviour patterns is a crucial factor in the identification of potential triggers, and can be used to anticipate future incidents.

Case example 4.1

An elderly woman suffering from dementia assaulted staff at irregular intervals. The incidents had no apparent cause, but she would become increasingly aroused before the assaults, and would appear angry. Only after several weeks did it become clear that the trigger to the assaults was the colour of clothing worn by visitors, staff, or other patients. The colour which upset her changed unpredictably over time, but knowing that particular colours upset the woman allowed staff at least to anticipate assaults, although not always to prevent them.

Limit setting

Limit setting is often a trigger for violent incidents, especially where limits are imposed and where restrictions on patient freedom are involved. In one study, Breakwell & Rowett (1989) found that 25% of violent incidents involved "the upholding of agency rules". Inconsistent limit setting has also been associated with an increased risk of aggression (Madden, 1977). Appropriate training in limit setting is important in reducing violence and in the avoidance of triggers (Infantino & Mustingo, 1985).

In setting limits staff may be seen by potential aggressors primarily as representatives of the 'system' rather than as individuals, particularly in settings where staff are in uniform. Hence the ability to 'personalise' oneself without loss of appropriate authority may be important (Turnbull *et al*, 1990). This can be done by the use of first names during a confrontation or the employment of any strategy which 'humanises' the participants, emphasising their individuality rather than their formal role, such as mentioning past activities with the client.

Presence of bystanders

Aggressive behaviour may be both triggered and reinforced by the actions of others. Staff may be required to control the behaviour of other clients, who may act as a 'chorus', encouraging the aggressor in the challenging behaviour. If another client has provided the trigger to the violence, or is the object of the violence, then removing him/her from the scene can be an effective intervention.

Breakwell (1989) suggests that audiences can be helpful in some situations, for example where help is required. She also notes the bystander phenomenon, where a number of clients or staff watch an assault without intervening. This response, described in several serious incidents, seems to result from a diffusion of responsibility for action in a large group (a solitary observer seems much more likely to intervene or to raise the alarm). This problem can best be tackled by addressing requests to specific people, for example "Helen, run and get help. Palvinder, take the other patents away", rather than a general "Help!".

It may be desirable to interview an aggressive person in a private office to ensure privacy and to minimise any encouragement and stimulation derived from an audience. However, as Coid discusses in Chapter 2, interviewing an angry or aggressive client alone with no easy means of summoning support is unwise. If aggressive clients are interviewed alone, it is important to be sure that other staff are aware of the interview, and that support is readily available.

Staff behaviour

When confrontations arise, the only element of the situation under the direct control of potential staff victims may well be their own immediate responses. The use of body language, verbal responses and other techniques is discussed in detail below, in the section on specific skills.

Arousal

Arousal is the last of the four components outlined above. It is the product of the cognitive and physiological changes produced within the organism in response to a perceived threat (some of the theoretical background is discussed in Chapter 1). These changes constitute an adaptive evolutionary response which gears the body for a primarily physical response to threat. These may involve *fight* responses, in which the threat is confronted, or *flight* responses, in which the threat is avoided.

These physiological responses may inhibit the ability to use the skills fundamental to effective communication, verbal de-escalation and problem solving. At low or optimal levels of stress there may be increased energy, concentration and motivation. At higher levels a series of maladaptive effects may impair motor skill and cognition, resulting in reductions in information-processing, decision-making and problem-solving ability (Dixon, 1987).

Enhanced arousal requires not only a triggering stimulus but a predisposition by the individual to label such an event as threatening. Novaco (1975, 1978) highlighted the relationship between such cognitive labelling and the subsequent development of anger and the person's predisposition towards violent behaviour. Novaco (1977) defines anger "as an emotional response to provocation, which is determined by a person's own unique cognitive, somatic-affective and behaviour patterns", and argues that external circumstances provoke anger only as mediated by their meaning to the individual.

There is compelling evidence of a relationship between overt expressions of anger, in the form of verbal abuse and threats (an expression of arousal), and the increased likelihood of the use of physical aggression (Breakwell & Rowett, 1989; McNeil & Binder, 1989). Not all episodes involving anger, verbal abuse or threatening behaviour precede or predict physical assault, but increased arousal is a major factor contributing to violent behaviour through its disinhibitory effects (Morton, 1986; Rice *et al*, 1990).

The specific behavioural indicators of arousal will vary between people and should, where possible, be interpreted in the context of an understanding of individual personality and normal baseline behaviour (Lanza, 1983). Knowledge of an individual's behavioural patterns are important elements in the prediction process, as this allows staff to identify changes from 'normal' or baseline behaviours, and acts as a key indicator of rising levels of arousal. Cues indicative of heightened arousal may, in turn, initiate heightened arousal in observers and lead to a self-reinforcing cycle, which may ultimately reduce the ability of all participants in an incident to employ constructive skills and strategies.

Information on the responses of confronted professionals (e.g. Rowett, 1986; Crane, 1986) suggests that many experience 'flight' responses. Another common response is the immobilisation or 'freezing' of the staff victim, who may make very few attempts at de-escalation or deflection of aggression.

Studies of violence-prone individuals (e.g. Toch, 1969) point to the significance of aggressive staff responses in the development of some violent incidents. These findings indicate the need for appropriate staff training in dealing with these incidents, using appropriate training models.

A *model of de-escalation*

Many staff develop considerable competence in the management of hostile behaviour through a combination of authority, confidence, sensitivity and experience. The difficulty lies in extrapolating such skills into a general code of guidance which can be applied to other settings and staff groups. For staff in the caring profession it is also important to recognise legal and ethical factors, and that the short-term demands of immediate safety may need to be balanced against longer-term expectations involving patient/client care and behavioural change.

Not all violent incidents are preventable. Some targeted staff, however, misread situational cues or use ineffective responses to violence from a client. Experience suggests that this is particularly so where the aggressor's behaviour is personally offensive or threatening. This may be because of increasing levels of arousal in both victim and aggressor, which result in enhanced threat perception, lowered rationality, and reduced responsiveness to conciliatory responses. This emphasises the need to base responses on an appreciation of arousal as an interactive and escalating cycle involving specific stages which may require different responses.

This section describes a systematic approach to de-escalation which addresses both the 'what' and the 'when' of effective staff responses. This approach also links with the therapeutic dimensions involving the promotion of alternative behaviour and provides a framework within which the policies and practice of the specific organisation can be applied. The main planks of the strategy are to maintain communication with the aggressor and to minimise factors which serve to promote or sustain arousal.

Within this conceptual framework we can outline a more systematic approach, involving:

    (a) a set of practice principles
    (b) a set of core interpersonal skills
    (c) a set of stage-specific response strategies.

The overall approach attempts to achieve a broad match between specific staff responses and the dominant emotions which are likely to shape an aggressor's behaviour at different levels of emotional arousal. It also attempts to ensure that such responses are consistent with the legal, ethical and value context in which the caring professions operate.

Practice principles

Challenging behaviour can be understood

Everyone has an absolute right to their feelings. Explore and try to understand the feelings and issues which promote the use of challenging or aggressive behaviour and try to help the person view these feelings more realistically.

Maintain self-esteem

Always try to maintain the safety and self-esteem of all participants in a confrontation. Do not try to 'win' or get into will struggles unless the situation requires the explicit exercise of authority. Do not defend situations which are the focus of an aggressor's resentment. Do not belittle or criticise aggressors even if they have lost control of themselves.

Attempt to maximise the choices open to an aggressor

Help aggressors to explore alternative solutions.

Respond early

Always try to intervene in developing situations at an early point to help to avoid further escalation.

Respond proportionately

Intervention should primarily represent an act of care. The response of staff should be based on an assessment of the degree of risk and the level of emotional arousal displayed by an aggressor. Staff behaviour should not exceed that of an aggressor in intensity. Where possible remain calm.

Address both short-term and longer-term goals

Where possible, staff should consider both short-term and long-term goals. An incident has not been truly resolved until this has been done.

Short term. Preservation of the safety and integrity of all present is the principle short-term goal.

Long term. Where possible, resolution of underlying difficulties and the promotion of alternative functional behaviours are the principle long-term goals.

In the context of the arousal cycle, the principle aim should be to help the aggressor move towards resolution of underlying difficulties while minimising the level of emotional arousal.

Develop awareness

While accepting your own limitations, attempt to develop awareness of key attitudes, behaviours and tolerances. Recognise the rights which we demand from others and our responsibility to respect theirs in turn.

Staff should attempt to recognise and change dysfunctional personal attitudes, which may include denial of risk or confrontational approaches.

Shared responsibility

Use the support available from others. The management of aggressive and violent behaviour in a professional setting is a shared responsibility, requiring action from the organisation, managers and staff. Safety and effective behaviour management should not be viewed as solely a matter of individual competence. The influence of the context of the interaction and the influence of an aggressor's prior learning should be recognised.

Be proactive

Ensure that the factors which may contribute to challenging behaviour, the way an incident should be managed and how participants should be supported afterwards are considered *before* an incident occurs.

Be realistic

Working with challenging behaviour can be very stressful. It is often the result of a person's long-term past difficulties. Where possible, responses to such behaviour should be part of a care plan. Be realistic in your expectations. Above all try not to take it personally! If assaulted, remember to forgive yourself.

Core interpersonal skills

Studies of the aetiology of aggression within health and welfare settings indicate the importance of staff attitudes and practices which serve to disempower or depersonalise an individual, reducing him/her to a 'problem' or set of symptoms (e.g. "the hernia in bed 6"). Enabling staff to develop skills and behaviours which promote patient/client individuality may be key factors in the maintenance of both therapeutic relationships and the avoidance of aggression. Recognised core skills include the following.

Empathy

Empathy is the ability both to understand the other person's viewpoint and feelings and to convey an accurate understanding of them to the person.

Respect

Convey interest and respect on the basis of a person's individuality and an active involvement in their situation.

Genuineness

Respond in a open, spontaneous and personalised manner which avoids stereotypes, institutionalised or 'over-professional' responses.

Concreteness

Deal with individuals, issues and feelings in concrete and specific terms which avoid vague, unspecific responses.

Integrity

Integrity is a complex notion. However, in this context it includes qualities such as: 'authority', in the sense of a confident awareness of one's competences and responsibilities; and 'fairness', the broad ability to assess problems from different perspectives and act within the constraints of 'justice' and 'altruism' or the general ability and motivation towards promoting the legitimate interests of others.

Specific skills

The above are individual qualities which should be recognised at the time of initial recruitment and developed by the process of professional training. They are conveyed and applied by a range of specific skills which have an observable behavioural component.

Communication skills

Effective communication is an interactive process involving both the accurate transmission and receipt of information while avoiding, for example, inattention and making assumptions which may diminish understanding of the other's position. During an aggressive confrontation there are additional priorities of active listening and the avoidance of any form of communication which heightens arousal, acts as a trigger or may be interpreted as a criticism or threat to the safety or self-esteem of the aggressor.

Non-verbal communication

Psychologists generally recognise non-verbal communication as the more powerful medium, with language mainly serving to convey detail (Mehrabian, 1969; Birdwhistell, 1971). In an aggressive encounter, key elements in effective non-verbal communication involve the avoidance of gestures which imply threat or dismissal, and ensuring consistency of the message conveyed at verbal and non-verbal levels. For instance, a verbal message of interest and concern may be undermined when delivered by staff with crossed arms and frowning expressions.

Posture, stance and eye contact are central to the non-verbal repertoire. In clinical situations clients may be confused or psychotic and have difficulty responding to verbal communication. Body posture should minimise threat and convey calm interest. Postures which involve standing facing an aggressor, the folding of arms across the chest or hands on hips can be interpreted as confrontational, and should be avoided. Standing at an angle to the subject with hands out of the pockets and held in an open posture is less threatening, and has the added advantage of decreasing the target area for an assault, and providing better balance. If possible, it is best to get both partners to a confrontation to sit, which may reduce the motivation to assault and provide staff with more time to anticipate potential physical assault.

Eye contact should be used carefully, and should simulate that of normal conversation. Prolonged eye contact may be interpreted as aggressive, while avoidance may be seen as demonstrating fear or lack of interest (Rice *et al*, 1990).

Invasion of personal space, sometimes involving extremely intimate contact, is often associated with the practice of both medicine and nursing, and the professions are allowed to transcend social norms relating to personal space and touch taboos. Physical intimacy is, however, subject to wide cultural variations, which require careful consideration. Generally an aggressor's intimate zone expands with rising arousal. There is considerable evidence linking the invasion of personal space beyond that considered acceptable with an increased risk of assaults, and that reducing infringements on personal space helps to reduce violent incidents (Negley & Manley, 1990).

In addition to an awareness that invasion of personal space is more likely to be designated as a latent 'threat' by aroused individuals, touch requires particular thought. Gertz (1980) reports the successful use of touch with highly distressed clients as part of a de-escalatory process, but only when staff were given permission. Bond (1982), however, describes the tendency for touch to be seen as patronising. Touch is also subject to complex social and sexual norms and taboos, and consideration should be given to the potential misinterpretation of touch and the vulnerability of staff to client complaints. Touching an aroused client therefore requires extreme caution. If it does seem appropriate, a gentle, slow approach after asking permission is best.

Verbal skills

In an aggressive encounter, staff ability to communicate effectively may determine the degree to which they are able both to understand the aggressor's underlying problems and motivations, and to avoid statements which are potentially provocative. Insulting or abusive language should obviously be avoided.

Breakwell (1989) also emphasises the need to avoid the use of 'barbs' – words or phases known to be provocative to the person concerned. Where barbs are not known, staff should carefully observe changes in the client's level of arousal during verbal interactions, and avoid repeating mistakes.

The use of clear, appropriate language at the level of the person's understanding and the appropriate timing of communication using simple, clear and uncomplicated questioning are important.

Questioning requires a person to consider and process the enquiry, and may help to maintain cognition rather than emotion as the principal determinant of behaviour, although sensitivity is required.

The tone of voice used requires thought. A quietly modulated tone is generally appropriate as it requires aroused subjects to listen actively to the staff member. Conversely, increasing the tone and volume of voice may convey authority and conviction, and an unexpected change in voice tone and volume or a loud shout can be an effective strategy in extreme situations. However, given the demands of privacy and the avoidance of further arousal, it is usually best to use the lowest volume consistent with clear communication.

Interest and an understanding of the problem can be enhanced by using open questions which avoid simple yes/no responses and invite the subject to explore or elaborate a point. 'Why' questions should be avoided because of their tendency to promote defensive answers. Understanding can also be increased by the use of paraphrasing, in which staff sum up their understanding of the person's statements in their own words. Rapport can be encouraged by the use of sustaining responses (e.g. "aha", "I see", "tell me more"), which encourage people to explore and elaborate their positions.

Davies (1989) proposes that in some instances it is preferable to 'mood match'. In conversation one normally matches the other's mood, but this convention is often disregarded when speaking to aggressive people (Argyle, 1983). The idea of mood matching is often misunderstood as meaning that staff should appear angry or annoyed, but this is not the case. Rather, the intention is to display concern, involvement or interest, and to demonstrate to the person that the importance of the issue is clearly appreciated and they are being taken seriously. Davies suggests that if arousal can be maintained at a level slightly less than that of the aggressor it may be possible to model a gradual reduction in arousal which induces a similar response. If this approach is used, it is important for the staff member to maintain some distance from the process in order to monitor the whole situation – so while expressing concern, they should still be monitoring their posture, closeness to an escape route, possible weapons which the aggressor could use, and so on.

Maintenance of self-control

Self-control rests upon self-understanding and an awareness of those situations which give rise to personal anxiety and the nature of one's likely responses. As Coid points out in Chapter 3, unexpected fear can be a valuable indicator to a staff member that something is amiss, even when there has been no obvious threat.

Constructive responses require that we attend to the 'voice of fear'. Although many people report enhanced clarity of thought and concentration during assaults, fear generally inhibits the cognitive processes, often producing a situation in which the body and the mind become locked and unresponsive. This can be partly overcome by an understanding of the process, and by the use of counteracting behavioural techniques. These can employ positive internal self-talk which stresses competence ("I can handle this constructively") and avoids the fostering of a victim mentality (e.g. "I can't cope, I am going to get hurt"). Any tendency for the body to lock into a static and rigid posture can be helped by the conscious bending of the knees and the lowering of the shoulders. Slow, steady diaphragmatic breathing will also help to modulate the physiological response and stave off panic reactions.

Assertiveness skills

Although assertiveness is frequently misunderstood as simply a means of getting one's own way, the concept offers a range of verbal strategies aimed at managing situations in a manner in which the self-esteem and integrity of both parties are preserved. Assertive responses contrast with aggressive and non-assertive or passive behaviours in which one party 'wins' at the expense of the other (Holland & Ward, 1990).

Wondrak (1989) recommends the use of five specific assertiveness techniques in the context of aggressive confrontations: side-stepping; self-disclosure; partial agreement; gentle confrontation; and being specific. These are dicussed in detail in textbooks on assertiveness.

In many situations, particularly those such as muggings, involving instrumental violence, the potential victim's refusal to submit may encourage the aggressor to assess the balance of advantage against risk and seek greener and less risky pastures. However, in other situations, such as sexual assault and rape, power and the wish to dominate and humiliate the victim may be a contributory motive, and so failure to concede may exacerbate the force used. As with all responses to aggression, the choice of response must depend directly on the judgement of the individual.

A systematic model of de-escalation

An aroused confrontation can be visualised as a process led by a pattern of changing and increasingly negative emotions in which an individual's rationality and potential responsiveness to conciliation progressively decreases, while their predisposition towards viewing the behaviour of others as threatening, and the potential for physically violent behaviour and the consequent risks to intervening staff, are progressively increased.

This emotional slope can be represented as a progress through broad stages dominated successively by anxiety, anger, and aggression, through to the emotional states underlying directly assaultive behaviours. A description of this curve is included in Chapter 1. Leadbetter's model, currently subject to evaluative research, is one way of bringing together these aspects in one approach, and is outlined below. Each stage requires a different focus of staff responses, which involve the employment of a range of specific tactics (Fig. 4.1).

Adopting a process model of de-escalation should assist in the appropriate matching of specific staff responses to the emotional needs of the aggressor. Although described sequentially, individuals enter the cycle at different levels of arousal. Indeed, many populations in care may be largely comprised of individuals for whom emotional lability or a heightened state of arousal and associated behaviours are habitual. Like other transition curves, such as loss, the progress of the individual along the curve is seldom smooth, and may involve switching between stages or fixation for prolonged periods in a particular stage. The overall aim of the staff response is to facilitate the subject's progress through successive stages, discussed under separate headings below, while minimising their ascent of the arousal slope.

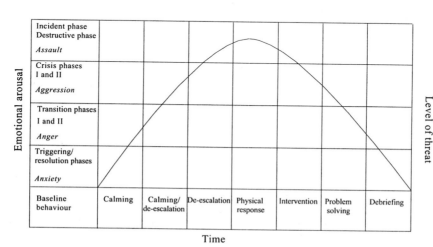

Fig. 4.1. Stages in a model of de-escalation

Stage 1. Triggering phase (*ascent*)

Dominant emotion – anxiety

The key initial indicator of the person's move away from normal, calm baseline behaviour will involve individual behaviours characteristic of anxiety. These may include agitation, pacing, and sighing, or inwardly directed behaviours such as withdrawal or avoidance of contact.

Staff response – calming

Aims

The aims here are:

(a) assessment of the subject's emotional state
(b) identification of the principal causal/triggering factors
(c) reduction of anxiety
(d) maintenance of verbal interaction/rapport
(e) problem solving (where possible).

Focus

The focus should be on:

(a) the subject's emotional state; this should be explored and acknowledged before any solutions are attempted
(b) the underlying problem.

Specific skills and qualities

Attending and communication skills are required, as are warmth, empathy, genuineness, active listening skills, and patience.

Potential tactics

Personalise yourself. This might involve the use of first names and, where possible, reminding the person of the strength of the relationship with the staff member and any positive action taken on their behalf in the past.

Paraphrasing. Restate the subject's perspectives in his/her own words to convey understanding and to encourage further reflection.

Feeling reflection. Correctly identify the person's feelings state ("You must have felt very sad when that happened").

Reassurance. Use praise and encouragement and confirm your willingness to help with the problem.

Open questions. Use of questions which invite further reflection as opposed to closed questions requiring a simple yes/no answer.

Programme involvement. Use of available activities or programmes to divert and occupy the person.

Things to avoid. Avoid inappropriate questions (e.g. "why" questions), which invite defensiveness; closed questions (yes/no), which inhibit problem exploration; complicated questions or the use of technical or inappropriate language. Likewise, avoid coercive advice, teaching, preaching, or statements which imply a judgement or criticism of the person. Avoid conveying threat, whether by condescending or authoritarian attitudes or by inappropriate non-verbal behaviour

Stage 2 – Transition phase (*ascent*)

Dominant emotion – anger

The onset of arousal may be triggered by events or interpretations in either the past or the present. The second stage denotes a shift towards hostile or negative perception of the present situation, although staff may not yet be the main focus of animosity or hostility.

Staff may therefore need to use aspects of both the preceding (triggering) stage, which is essentially person focused, and the following (crisis) stage, which is more concerned with the containment of behaviour.

Staff response – calming/de-escalation

See Stage 3, below.

Stage 3 – Crisis phase (*ascent*)

As arousal increases, the subject's anger may become focused upon intervening staff or others in the area. The likelihood of the person interpreting the actions of others as threatening is often increased, with a corresponding reduction in willingness to respond to conciliatory behaviour. Judgement, reasoning and problem-solving abilities still maintain some influence on behaviour, however, and this crisis phase may constitute a watershed which will determine whether the aggressor progresses towards the use of overtly violent behaviour or responds to the interventions of staff.

Given reducing rationality (the willingness to pursue actions consistent with self-interest), the potential to resolve any underlying grievance by rational discussion is likely to decline and the focus of staff intervention may have to shift towards the containment of behaviour rather than problem solving.

Dominant emotion – aggression

An explicit level of threat to responding staff may emerge at this stage. Indicators may include poor impulse control, agitation, and threatening gestures, including finger pointing, raised fists, invasion of personal space or verbal abuse and profanity, or shouting.

Staff response – de-escalation

Aims

The aim here is:

(a) to prevent further escalation and possible violence
(b) the active reduction of the level of the client's arousal
(c) to assist the client in re-engaging cognition to replace emotion as a primary drive in determining behaviour
(d) to attempt to restructure the client's cognitions away from thoughts linked to anger
(e) to maintain the safety and integrity of all present.

Focus

The increased potential for violent behaviour requires that concern with the aggressor's agenda is replaced by the management of risk as a principle focus of staff response. This will involve:

(a) the preparation and coordination of supportive staff members; incidents can, however, arise very quickly, and as this may not always be possible, effective coordination requires proactive incident drills
(b) the removal of bystanders who may reinforce aggression and prevent or complicate the resolution of the incident
(c) the removal (discretely) of possible weapons
(d) the containment of significant threatening behaviour.

Potential tactics

Maintain verbal communication, while allowing silence where it appears helpful.

Avoid the loss of authority and attempt to minimise the sense of power which the employment of aggression often confers on aggressors. Avoid making major concessions on substantive issues, but allow simpler concessions where possible ("I can't do anything about you being detained under the section, but I can call your wife to let her know how you feel").

Request direct compliance with staff requests. Warning the person of the possible consequences and outcomes of the behaviour will be more useful than the use of threats, ultimatums or overt coercion, which may reinforce aggression or act as triggers. Allow the aggressor time for reflection. A clear indication of the unacceptability of specific behaviours may be required ("Being in hospital doesn't mean it's all right for you to hit anyone").

Attempt to encourage the aggressor into a positive pattern of responses. This can be done by requesting small concessions which can be accepted before requesting any major concessions ("the little to large principle").

Use self-disclosure (common experiences, shared problems, etc.).

Build alliances or agree with legitimate criticisms where this is merited ("You are right, we should have told you earlier that you were being moved to a different unit"). Presenting other perspectives of the situation may be useful, but do not try to argue or coerce agreement. Avoid contradictions and responses which involve specifically yes/no answers.

Use conditional limit setting (e.g. "Once you have stopped shouting we will resolve the issue").

Mood match (avoiding aggression – see page 60).

Use distraction/diversion.

Use time-out/delayed compliance ("Why don't we come back to this in ten minutes", etc.).

Stage 4 – Destructive phase (*summit*)

Staff response – physical response (escape; self-defence; physical restraint)

Aims

The aim here is to preserve the physical safety of all participants.

Focus

As the aggressor's arousal peaks, reduced impulse control can result in physical aggression towards people or objects. Continued verbal negotiation becomes futile. Risks to the physical welfare of client, staff and bystanders may become dependent on an adequate physical staff response in the form of escape, self-defence or physical restraint. The action taken will depend on a judgement of the level of risk involved in specific actions and the responsibility carried by staff for others in the situation. Flight rather than fight responses are generally best. In some very high-risk situations, such as hostage incidents where a weapon is being used, or where furniture is being destroyed but intervention could lead to greater danger to patients or staff, it may be necessary to comply with commands from the aggressor. Hostage incidents are discussed briefly later in the chapter. This stage marks a summit, after which arousal levels will reduce, whether in response to staff action or physical exhaustion.

Specific skills

   (a) risk assessment
   (b) 'breakaway' and physical restraint skills (see later)
   (c) staff coordination skills.

Stage 5 – Descent phase

Dominant emotion – aggression

Staff response – intervention

This stage commences with the cessation of overtly destructive behaviour. The person's level of arousal may visibly reduce, although the physiological and cognitive changes induced by arousal will maintain a heightened perception of threat, which may result in fresh violent behaviour in response to inadvertent triggers. Staff must remain vigilant. This stage is a second period of potential crisis.

Aims

The aim here is the resumption of staff control over the immediate situation and the continuing monitoring and containment of risk.

Focus

The nature of staff responses during this stage will be determined by the context of the incident and operational practices. Containment of risk may require that additional staff, police or security personnel are summoned and coordinated.

   In some settings chemical sedation may be administered.

In institutional or care settings the routines and policies of the unit will decide specific staff actions during this stage. These may include the use of seclusion or safe alternative activities which assist or continue the calming process. However, no aggressor should be returned to communal activities until staff are satisfied that a sufficiently reduced level of arousal has been attained.

Specific skills

Staff/activity coordination skills.

Stage 6 – Transition phase (*descent*)

Dominant emotion – anger

Staff response – problem solving

The immediate risk of physical injury to others should diminish during this stage, which acts as a bridge between the short-term management of an incident in which safety is the over-riding aim, and the longer-term aim of reducing the likelihood of the recurrent use of aggressive behaviours by the promotion of insight and the development of alternative behaviours.

Aims

The aim here is:

(a) to maximise staff control of the immediate situation
(b) to minimise the sense of power produced by the use of aggression on the part of the subject
(c) to resolve (where possible) underlying problems or trigger issues
(d) to prepare the person for the resolution phase
(e) to clarify staff expectations of the person's immediate behaviour
(f) to apply sanctions (where needed).

Focus

With the continuing reduction in arousal levels and consequent increased levels of rationality, staff may no longer be the primary focus for the aggressor's negative feelings, and functional behaviours may gradually return. This stage is a further period of transition between focused aggression and other emotions. Increased rationality may allow resumed attempts by staff to explore underlying difficulties, and the ability to engage constructively with staff attempts to resolve underlying triggering issues should also increase. The imposition of punishments or sanctions on unacceptable behaviour are less likely to act as triggers for resumed aggression when employed at this stage.

Specific skills

Intervention techniques may be categorised under three principal headings:

(a) behavioural modification approaches which employ the use of sanctions or rewards, or involvement in valued or aversive activities
(b) counselling approaches involving the promotion of insight
(c) problem solving approaches involving
    (i) indirect approaches aimed at helping the subject identify available options and alternatives, or
    (ii) direct approaches involving the provision of advice, information, and so on.

These may be used singly or in combination.

Stage 7 – Resolution phase (*post-incident*)

Dominant emotions – anger, possible guilt, remorse, resentment

While safety and the containment of aggressive behaviour are always principal concerns, the promotion of functional social behaviours is a further area of responsibility in most care and clinical settings.

Involvement in a violent incident usually generates powerful and often primitive emotions for all concerned. Guilt, concern at possible performance failure and feelings of retribution or anger are common responses. These can complicate the manner in which an incident is handled once the immediate risk is past, and they detract from the opportunity which an incident of aggressive behaviour affords for the promotion of new learning and coping skills for all participants. (Brehaut & Darby, 1992).

Not all violent incidents constitute a crisis for those involved. The term is best applied to situations in which a person has attempted to employ his/her normal repertoire of coping skills without success. Consequently, while a violent event certainly constitutes a 'problem' for staff, it also contains elements of 'opportunity'. In the aftermath of a period of substantially heightened arousal the aggressive individual is likely to experience a range of emotions, physical symptoms and altered cognitions. Common feelings include depression, physical exhaustion, disorientation, contrition, inability to perform practical tasks and reduced sequential memory. It is important to remember that such factors are likely to influence the behaviour and affect of both the aggressor and staff involved in critical incidents.

This holds important implications for the ability of the staff involved to continue to function effectively or assist in the subsequent management of the aggressor. The effect on sequential memory and cognitive ability should be acknowledged by managers, who may have potentially conflicting responsibilities for staff care, responsibilities for the assailant, and investigation of the incident. Staff debriefing after a serious incident is discussed further in Chapter 6, while post-incident support for staff is reviewed in Chapter 7.

Staff response

The focus of staff response should now shift from the containment and management of the critical incident to the attempt to help the aggressor develop insight into the causes, triggers, processes, behaviours and consequences of his/her involvement. This is attempted by means of some form of debriefing interview. Judgement is required on how this is best conducted, but aims should include:

    (a) to promote personal learning/growth
    (b) to facilitate the development of the functional behaviours
    (c) to facilitate the reintroduction of the subject into the unit regimen.

Aims

A debriefing interview aims to help the aggressor develop insight into the causes of aggressive behaviour and the development of adaptive alternative behaviour patterns. This may require staff to suspend judgements about the 'rights or wrongs' of the incident and conduct the interview in a patient and non-threatening manner.

It is advisable for the interview to proceed through specific stages. At each stage the interviewer attempts to help the subject understand how each stage informs the next. The interviewer should first attempt to explore the aggressor's perception and interpretation of the issue before offering any alternative perceptions and interpretations available from other sources.

The successive stages can be presented alphabetically:

(a) *antecedents* – the exploration of the factors which contributed to or triggered the aggressive incident. Particular attention should be paid to identifiable triggers, the aggressor's cognitions and interpretations and their influence on his/her observable behaviour

(b) *behaviour* – the detailed exploration of the aggressor's resulting behaviour

(c) *consequences* – the consequences which resulted from the behaviour:
   (i)   for the participant
   (ii) for others.

(d) *design* – the interviewer should attempt to design a plan to aid the aggressor in the avoidance of the recurrence of the behaviour identified. The plan should include:
   (i)   the circumstances or situations in which the behaviour is likely to recur
   (ii) the alternative behaviours which the aggressor could attempt to employ
   (iii) the help which will be available to the participant (e.g. staff support)
   (iv) the consequences which will result from the recurrence of the dysfunctional behaviour identified and the rewards which will result from the employment of alternative functional behaviours.

(e) *enter* – the interviewer should assist the aggressor in entering back into the routine of the unit.

Focus

The principal focus of staff interest is to create a safe, supportive environment which will free the aggressor to explore underlying behaviours and cognitions. Additionally, aggressive incidents may be a source of considerable interest and entertainment within a peer group. It may be necessary therefore to ease the aggressor's reintroduction into the normal routine.

Maximising the constructive potential of an aggressive incident will involve the following.

(a) *Selection of interviewer.* An appropriate staff member must be selected to conduct the debriefing interview; staff with a positive relationship with the aggressor may be appropriate.

However, where such staff have been involved in the incident such a personal involvement may be best avoided.

(b) *Site of the interview.* A room or office which provides privacy and freedom from interruption will assist the exploration and disclosure process. However, this has to be balanced by the need to ensure the safety of interviewing staff against the possible resumption of aggression.

(c) *Appropriate timing.* An accurate assessment of the aggressor's ability to discuss the incident is required. Interviews conducted immediately after an incident may lead to the preoccupation of the aggressor with causal factors and injustice. However, it is advisable for interviews to be conducted at the earliest reasonable point following an incident.

Physical responses to aggression

Despite the strategies for preventing violence discussed in this volume – personal, medical and organisational – violent incidents will continue to take place. Professional practice requires the recognition that assaults are, to a degree, inevitable and that it is therefore incumbent upon professionals to take steps to prepare themselves adequately (Whitman *et al*, 1976). Although many professional staff believe they can 'handle themselves' in a violent incident despite having had no relevant training, the practice of untrained staff may be shambolic, ineffective, seriously unsafe and legally questionable (Paterson *et al*, 1992).

Tarbuck (1992*a*) notes that the consideration or application of force must always be considered an extremely serious matter, "abhorrent to the professional" and acceptable only when demonstrably a last resort. The practice must be subject to rigorous professional scrutiny designed to promote good practice and pre-empt or eliminate abuse. In applying physical intervention techniques, professionals must be aware of the complex legal and ethical boundaries of practice. These may vary between professions, settings and nationalities (Miller, 1991; Tarbuck, 1992*b*). These issues are discussed further in Chapter 8.

Although generally commissioned in the wake of an incident involving serious injury or a fatality, a number of reports from official and professional bodies have called for the adoption of a specific and systematic approach to physical restraint and staff training (e.g. Department of Health and Social Security, 1988; British Association of Social Workers, 1988; Department of Health, 1993). Despite this, many professions have failed to develop or provide training in physical responses, the very skills potentially of most value to staff in extreme situations. Often guidance is framed in general terms and fails to offer staff sufficient practical advice on safe intervention. Staff consequently frequently feel unsupported, tending to view such guidance as an agency 'back covering' exercise, aimed at limiting liability. Staff may consequently be more certain of what they cannot do and less certain of what they can do. This neglect is also likely to perpetuate gender-based practices such as the reliance on men in situations requiring physical intervention. This may provide a model to aggressors which equates competence and authority with masculinity and physical size, effectively suggesting 'might is right', as well as effectively disempowering women staff, who are likely to constitute the majority of the workforce in most health and care settings.

Although the research literature on staff training in physical response techniques is disappointingly scant, it confirms a clear need for training in the physical management of aggression and violence (Health Services Advisory Committee, 1987). The need for staff training has also been emphasised by the Mental Welfare Commission in Scotland (1994). Such training needs to be offered as part of an integrated programme whose curriculum includes theories of aggression, triggers and high-risk situations, and de-escalation techniques, rather than a free-standing course which courts the risk of promoting the perception of physical response as a strategy of first resort (Robinson & Barnes, 1989). Integrated programmes have been associated with subsequent decreases in violent incidents and injuries to staff and clients.

Lack of comparative evaluative research in this area makes it difficult to choose between competing strategies. A wide variety of programmes and specific approaches to physical responses have been described (Infantino & Mustingo, 1985; MacDonnell *et al*, 1991), including approaches described as therapeutic holding (Barlow, 1989), therapeutic crisis intervention (Badlong *et al*, 1992) and control and restraint (Paterson *et al*, 1992; Gilbert, 1988). Perhaps the best known of these approaches is 'control and restraint' training, which was developed originally within the Home Office for use by uniformed public sector staff. It offers a variety of individual and team approaches to physical restraint, in addition to 'minimum force' breakaway techniques aimed at assisting a potential victim to escape from a physical assault. It also aims to offer a 'gender free' system, in which competence is based on technique rather than size. It has received official endorsement by a number of professional bodies, including psychiatric nursing. However, the use of the physical restraint techniques within residential social work has become the focus of significant controversy (e.g. Social Services Inspectorate and Department of Health, 1993).

In the context of the Community Care reforms, many staff groups are reporting increasing difficulties in coping with the more extreme forms of client behaviour which may previously have been managed more effectively in contained settings. The growing recognition of staff risk and employer liability has fostered a vocal lobby for the development of more professional and systematic responses to aggression management. The hoped for solution has tended towards an official endorsement of specific methods of restraint by government which would provide a 'gold standard' and resolve the dilemma of individual organisations. However, given recent decisions in the care sector, such formal 'official' approval seems unlikely. The responsibility therefore remains on individual organisations and managers to evaluate and select an approach to physical restraint and breakaway training which will meet their specific needs.

No system can guarantee compete safety. Some approaches are the product of careful development. Others may give more specific cause for concern. Many have been developed in cultural or operational contexts which do not translate well to other settings. Within the current market context of training provision, the range of competing commercial providers and the lack of systematic, independent evaluation of approaches suggests that care should be taken in evaluating different systems before selecting an approach upon which to base a training strategy.

Before describing a number of the most simple and common 'breakaway' techniques drawn from the control and restraint system, it must be emphasised that such written descriptions in themselves do not produce adequate competence and may tempt the unwise into the dangers of false confidence. Safe and consistent staff practice can be developed only through participation in an integrated training programme on violence management in which specific approaches to physical escape and restraint are taught by competent, accredited instructors. This should be done in the context of a training strategy which provides adequate opportunities for revision and call-back training and which ensures that staff practice conforms to approved guidance, maintains competence and avoids skill decay.

Proficiency cannot be gained from reading the text alone. Seek training from a qualified instructor and practice under expert supervision before attempting to apply any of these techniques.

It is neither possible nor desirable to give a comprehensive overview of all the available techniques, which could occupy another book as large as the present volume. Readers interested in further training should contact their respective professional organisations for details of reputable programmes and trainers.

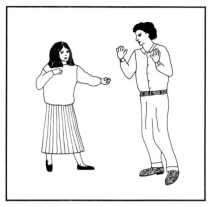

Fig. 4.2. Stance   Fig. 4.3. Wrist grab

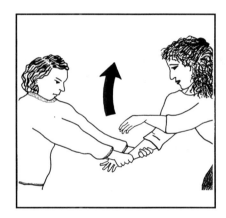

Fig. 4.4. Two-handed wrist grab   Fig. 4.5. Hair grab

Remember:

    (a) do not freeze if attacked; do something – shout, scream, use an alarm if available, run away

    (b) if you use a technique, do it quickly, do it with force, and get out of the situation.

Stance

The importance of posture has already been discussed. When talking to an upset client it is important to adopt a stance that will afford some protection if you are assaulted. Stand slightly sideways, holding the arms in a position where they could be used to block a blow (Fig. 4.2). Have as relaxed a manner as possible. Maintain discreet eye contact at all times.

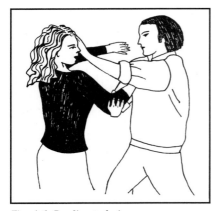

Fig. 4.6. Bowling technique

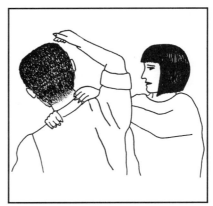

Fig. 4.7. Strangle push–pull

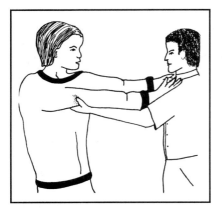

Fig. 4.8. Pinch on upper arm

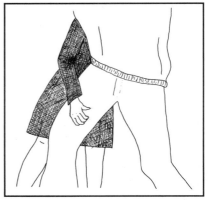

Fig. 4.9. Pinch on thigh

Grabbing

Wrist grabs and escape procedures are shown in Figs 4.3 and 4.4. The idea is to pull against the thumb, which is the weakest part of the grip.

Hair grabs

If grabbed by the hair, the natural reaction is to attempt to prise an attacker's fingers loose. This tends to be both ineffective and painful. A more effective response is to bring your own hands up over your head, clench them together and push down on top of the attacker's knuckles as hard as you can. If attacked from the front, bend forwards and step back while continuing to press hard. If attacked from the rear, step sideways and then backwards, maintaining the pressure on the assailant's knuckles (Fig. 4.5).

Bowling technique

If attacked from the front, adopt the defensive stance by moving your left leg backwards, moving to a position where you are side on to your assailant. At the same time, swing your right hand over the assailant's hand as if bowling overhand and turning your body. The procedure, although complex to describe, is easy to execute (Fig. 4.6).

Strangle grab

If grabbed from in front (Fig. 4.7), reach under the attacker's arm and grasp the elbow, pulling down sharply. With your free hand place your forefinger under your attacker's nose and push back firmly. This should turn the assailant, enabling you to escape.

Pinch releases

The idea of the pinch is to grasp the attacker's skin or muscle and nip or pinch sharply. The pinch can be applied to the triceps area or to the inner and upper aspect of the thigh (Figs 4.8 and 4.9).

Pressure can also be applied to the assailant's sternum. Place a knuckle on the sternum and push hard while twisting. Do not use a punch to initiate the move, as severe injury can result.

Pinches can be used in a variety of situations, for example in a strangle hold, or if grasped in a bear hug from in front or behind.

These latter techniques should be used with caution, as they involve the use of pain and, if unsuccesful, could inflame an already dangerous situation.

Hostage situations

Hostage taking is well recognised within penal settings and during terrorist incidents. In the caring professions there is a range of situations in which staff may be unwillingly detained by explicit coercion or implied threat (Turner, 1984*a*; Norris, 1990). The difficulty in identifying the frequency of these incidents in care settings indicates the absence of standardised or centralised recording systems and the lack of systematic research in this area (Turner, 1984*b*).

TABLE 4.1
Hostage incident stages/responses

Stage	Possible reactions	Desired actions
Alarm Initiation of hostage situation	Extreme fear, panic, shock, denial	Implement a pre-learned response strategy – act to relax yourself – do not act precipitously by resisting, particularly if weapons are involved. Comply quietly with instructions
Crisis Continuance of situation after initiation	Denial	Act to carry out normal role, e.g. if doctor or nurse tend to sick if circumstances permit. Continue to comply quietly. Do not draw attention to self unless absolutely necessary
Accommodation Prolonged captivity	Boredom claustrophobia, stress, 'Stockholm syndrome'	Identify self as person rather than a 'faceless' hostage. Establish relationship with captor(s)
Resolution End of situation	Exhaustion, relief, confusion	Acceptance of help/support. Comply with instructions of intervention agencies
After incident After release	Post-trauma anxiety/ disorder	Seek skilled help early

Adapted from Strentz (1984)

In conjunction with aggression management in general, the possibility of hostage-taking incidents requires consideration and planning within the context of agency policy, guidelines and effective research (Powell, 1991; Rahe & Geneder, 1992), as training in coping strategies for potential victims of hostage-taking incidents can improve their ability to deal with such situations (Moore, 1986).

In a careful analysis of hostage incidents, Strentz (1979) suggests that victims go through an adaptive process involving four specific stages. These are outlined in Table 4.1, together with a summary of possible reactions and advice on effective responses.

Different hostage incidents vary in relation to the level of threatened or actual violence, the motivation of the hostage takers, the numbers held, and the location and duration of the incident (Turner, 1984c). The personality characteristics of both hostages and hostage takers, which are important factors, also vary from incident to incident.

Fields (1980) describes four basic threats commonly used in hostage situations: the threat to life, the threat to bodily integrity, the threat to security, and the threat to self-image. These can combine and contribute to the experience of extreme fear, panic and a profound sense of powerlessness in victims. The hostage needs to be able to mobilise existing coping strategies and potential new coping skills in order to survive the experience (Macduff, 1992).

Similarities exist between effective de-escalation techniques and responses appropriate to hostage incidents (Rice *et al*, 1990). Self-awareness and the carefully applied use of self are integral to successful practice in both areas. Tardiff (1989) suggests that the giving of instructions and negotiation can be effective, given skill and sensitivity to the reaction of the hostage takers. Many authors, however, recommend 'quiet compliance' in hostage situations, given the priority of physical safety (Powell, 1991).

A significant and widely recognised victim response centres on the 'Stockholm syndrome' (Strentz, 1979). This comprises:

(a) development of positive feelings towards captors by those being held
(b) development of negative feelings by captives towards representatives of authority or external agencies
(c) development by captors of positive feelings towards those they are holding captive.

It involves the paradoxical development of positive emotional bonds between captives and captors. Although a complex phenomenon, the 'Stockholm syndrome' may be the result of captives identifying with the power and authority imposed by the hostage takers on their immediate situation and the consequent reduction of identification with legitimate authority, whose ability actively to ensure hostage safety may seem more remote.

Even after very brief periods of captivity, victims may experience serious psychological consequences which can require the provision of skilled help to assist recovery and promote readjustment.

Conclusions

There is no easy answer to the problems posed by the use of aggression and violence towards health and welfare staff. Self-awareness fostered and promoted by active training and adequate policy initiatives are fundamental. Staff need to avoid complacency and develop a balanced awareness of the risks and potentially effective responses. Above all, the avoidance of inappropriate self-blame and open discussion with colleagues are fundamental to the maintenance of coping skills.

Summary points

- Individualising the problem of violence to staff interferes with a coordinated organisational response. Teaching of de-escalation and physical skills can only be effective if it is part of an organisational strategy.
- Assaults require a victim, a weapon (which can be a fist), a trigger and a state of arousal. Become aware of common triggers, such as limit setting, and take extra care. Monitoring a person's state of arousal should be a habit.
- De-escalation involves the use of verbal and non-verbal techniques to reduce hostility and likelihood of assault. The techniques cannot be applied at random: alter the approach depending on the state of arousal of the potential assailant. Many staff continue to try to calm agitated people long after they should have left to seek extra help. Your priorities in a violent situation should be the safety of yourself and others.
- Monitor your own reactions in a threatening situation. Stay as calm as possible, and assess the situation, including possible escape routes. If there are bystanders, consider whether you should ask them to get help. Be specific in your requests. Do not be afraid to leave if that seems the best strategy. You do not need to 'win' the confrontation.
- Physical breakaway skills can be life saving. If you are likely to need to use them, seek appropriate training as soon as possible. Practise them as often as you can.
- In the post-incident phase consider who should review the incident with the assailant, and what lessons can be learned from it. Make sure other staff know of any potential for violence.
- In hostage situations 'quiet compliance' is probably the best tactic, but in longer episodes, personalising yourself to the captor is often worthwhile.

A systematic model of de-escalation

Phase 1. Triggering
- Dominant emotion: anxiety
- Staff response: calming
- Key points: demonstrate interest, problem solve, acknowledge and explore feelings, use counselling skills

Phase 2. Transition
- Dominant emotion: rising anger
- Staff response: calming/de-escalation
- Key points: as Phase 1 plus those from Phase 3, manage space – give distance; do not match anger with anger; avoid provocation; keep talking – set limits and give directions; be prepared to negotiate compromise; explore consequences; use assertiveness skills; personalise self; get assistance

Phase 3. Crisis
- Dominant emotion: increasing anger and aggression
- Staff response: de-escalation
- Key points: as Phase 2, plus avoid unrealistic problem solving /feeling exploration; increase space; warn of consequences (do not threaten); be prepared to withdraw and seek assistance; try to maintain communication

Phase 4. Destructive behaviour (summit)
- Dominant behaviour: assault/destruction
- Staff response: escape/defend/restrain (compliance if very high risk situation)

Phase 5. Descent phase
- Dominant emotion: decreasing anger and aggression
- Staff response: focused management
- Key points: monitor aggressor's arousal level carefully; avoid reigniting aggression; contain situation; ensure continuing assistance of staff and/or police; avoid retaliation or revenge; be patient

Phase 6. Transition (descent)
- Dominant feelings: decreasing anger/anxiety
- Key points: resume focus on problem solving/feelings; impose sanctions (if appropriate)

References

ARGYLE, M. (1983) *The Psychology of Interpersonal Behaviour.* London: Penguin.

BADLONG, M., HOLDEN, M. & MOONEY, A. (1992) *National Residential Childcare Project Therapeutic Crisis Intervention.* Family Life Development Centre, College of Human Ecology, Cornell University.

BAILEY, R. H. (1977) *Violence and Aggression.* The Netherlands (B.V.): Time-Life.

BARLOW, D. J. (1989) Therapeutic holding: effective intervention with the aggressive child. *Journal of Psychosocial Nursing and Mental Health Services,* **27**, 10–14.

BIRDWHISTELL, R. L. (1971) *Kinesics and Context.* London: Allen Lane.

BOND, M. (1982) Dare you say "no". *Nursing Mirror,* **13**, October, 40–42.

BREAKWELL, G. (1989) *Facing Physical Violence.* Leicester/London: British Psychological Society/Routledge.

—— & Rowett, C. (1989) Violence and social work. In *Human Aggression, Naturalistic Approaches* (eds J. Archer & K. Browne). London: Routledge.

BREHAUT, R. & DARBY, K. (1992) A red rag to a bull. *Community Care,* 5 March, 18–20.

BRITISH ASSOCIATION OF SOCIAL WORKERS (1988) *Violence to Social Workers.* Birmingham: British Association of Social Workers.

BROWN, R., BUTE, S. & FORD, P. (1986) *Social Workers at Risk: The Prevention and Management of Violence.* London: MacMillan.

CRANE, D. (1986) *Violence on Social Workers. University of East Anglia, Social Work Monograph 46.* Norwich: University of East Anglia.

DAVIES, W. (1989) The prevention of assault on professional helpers. In *Clinical Approaches to Violence* (eds K. Howell & C. R. Hollis). pp 311-329. Chichester: Wiley.

DEPARTMENT OF HEALTH (1993) *Permissible Forms of Control in Children's Residential Care* (LAC (93) 13). London: HMSO.

DEPARTMENT OF HEALTH AND SOCIAL SECURITY (1988) *Report of the DHSS Advisory Committee on Violence to Staff.* Chairperson: Lord Skelmersdale. London: HMSO.

DIXON, N. F. (1987) *Our Own Worst Enemy.* London: Futura.

FIELDS, M. (1980) Victims of terrorism: the effects of prolonged stress. *Evaluation and Change* , special issue, pp 76–83.

GERTZ, B. (1980) Training for prevention of assaultive behaviour in a psychiatric setting. *Hospital and Community Psychiatry,* **31**, 628–630.

GILBERT, J. (1988) Exercising some restraint. *Social Work Today,* October, 16–18.

HEALTH SERVICES ADVISORY COMMITTEE (1987) *Violence to Staff in the Health Services.* London: Health and Safety Executive.

HOLLAND, S. & WARD, C. (1990) *Assertiveness – A Practical Approach.* Bicester-Oxon: Winslow Press.

INFANTINO, J. A. & MUSTINGO, S. (1985) Assaults and injuries among staff with and without training in aggression control techniques. *Hospital and Community Psychiatry,* **36**, 1312–1314.

JOHNSTONE, S. (1988) Guidelines for social workers coping with violent clients. *British Journal of Social Work,* **18**, 377–390.

LANZA, M. L. (1983) Reactions of the nursing staff to physical assault. *Hospital and Community Psychiatry,* **34**, 44–47.

LEADBETTER, D. (1993*a*) *Systematic De-escalation of Aggression: An Approach to Risk Management and Behavioural Change for Health and Welfare Staff.* Lothian Regional Council Social Work Department In-Service Training Programme Training Support Brochure.

—— (1993*b*) Assaults on social work staff: the experience of one Scottish department. *British Journal of Social Work,* **23**, 613–628.

—— & PHILLIPS, R. (1990) Violent sessions in the classroom. *Social Work Today,* 1 February.

LION, J. R., SNYDER, W. & MERRILL, G. L. (1981) Under-reporting of assaults in a state hospital. *Hospital and Community Psychiatry*, **32**, 497–498.

MacDonnell, A., Dearden, B. & Richens, A. (1991) Staff training in the management of violence and aggression: 1. Setting up a training system. *Mental Handicap*, **19**, 73–76.

Macduff, D. R. (1992) Social issues in the management of released hostages. *Hospital and Community Psychiatry*, **43**, 825–828.

Madden, D. J. (1977) Voluntary and involuntary treatment of aggressive patients. *American Journal of Psychiatry*, **134**, 553–555.

McNeil, D. E. & Binder, R. L. (1989) Relationship between pre-admission threats and later violent behaviour by acute psychiatric inpatients. *Hospital and Community Psychiatry*, **40**, 605–608.

Mehrabian, A. (1969) *Tactics in Social Influence*. New Jersey: Prentice-Hall.

Mental Welfare Commission (1994) *Annual Report 1993*. Edinburgh: Mental Welfare Commission.

Miller, R. (1991) Hitting back. *Nursing Times*, **87**, 56–58.

Moore, J. D. (1986) Spokanes Robbery Education Programme. *FBI Law Enforcement Bulletin*, **49**, 11.

Morton, P. (1986) Managing assault: your patient is losing control and you're a convenient target. *American Journal of Nursing*, October, **86**, 1114–1116.

National Union of Public Employees (1991) Violence in the NHS. *Health Service News*, 9 April.

Negley, E. N. & Manley, J. T. (1990) Environmental interventions in assaultive behaviour. *Journal of Gerontological Nursing*, **16**, 29–32.

Norris, D. (1990) *Violence Against Social Workers: The Implications for Practice*. London: Jessica Kingsley.

Novaco, R. W. (1975) A*nger Control: The Development and Evaluation of an Experimental Treatment*. Lexington: DC Health Co.

—— (1976) The function and regulation of the arousal of anger. *American Journal of Psychiatry*, **133**, 1124–1128.

—— (1977) Stress inoculation: a cognitive therapy for anger and its application to a case of depression. *Journal of Consulting and Clinical Psychology*, **45**, 600–608.

—— (1978) Anger and coping with stress. In *Cognitive Behaviour Therapy* (eds J. P. Foreyt & D. P. Rathjen). New York: Penguin.

Paterson, B., Turnbull, J. & Aitken, I. (1992) An evaluation of a training course in the short term management of aggression. *Nurse Education Today*, **12**, 368–375.

Powell, M. K. (1991) Hostage situation policy statement for the emergency department. *Journal of Emergency Nursing*, **17**, 313–314.

Rahe, R. H. & Geneder, E. (1992) Adaptation to and recovery from captivity stress. *Military Medicine*, **148**, 577–585.

Rice, M., Harris, G. L., Varney, G., *et al* (1990) *Violence in Institutions: Understanding, Prevention and Control*. Ontario: Mental Health Centre, Penetangusihene.

Robinson, S. & Barnes, C. (1989) Continuing education in relation to the prevention and management of violence. In *Directions in Nursing Research* (eds J. Wilson Barnett & S. Robinson). London: Scutar Press.

Rowett, C. (1986) *Violence in Social Work*. Cambridge: Institute of Criminology.

Siann, G. (1985) *Accounting for Aggression: Perspectives ion Aggression and Violence*. London: George Allen and Unwin.

Social Services Inspectorate and the Department of Health (1993) *A Place Apart: An Investigation into the Handling and Outcome of Serious Injuries to Children and Other Matters at Aycliffe Centre for Children, County Durham*. London: SSI.

Stark, C. & Kidd, B. (1992) Violence and junior doctors working in psychiatry. *Psychiatric Bulletin*, **16**, 144–145.

Steadman, H. J. (1982) A situational approach to violence. *International Journal of Law and Psychiatry*, **5**, 171–186.

STEVENSON, S. (1991) Heading off aggression with verbal de-escalation. *Journal of Psychosocial Nursing*, **29**, 6–10.

STRENTZ, T. (1979) The Stockholm syndrome: law enforcement policy and ego defences of the hostage. *FBI Law Enforcement Bulletin*, **48**, 2–12.

—— (1984) Hostage survival guidelines. In *Violence in the Medical Care Setting: a Survival Guide* (ed. J. Turner). Colorado: Aspen.

TARBUCK, P. (1992*a*) Use and abuse of control and restraint. *Nursing Standard*, **6**, 30–33.

—— (1992*b*) Ethical standards and human rights. *Nursing Standard*, **3**, 27–36.

TARDIFF, K. (1989) *Assessment and Management of Violent Patients*. London: American Psychiatric Press.

TOCH, H. (1969) *Violent Men: An Inquiry into the Psychology of Violence*. Chicago: Aldine.

TURNBULL, J., AITKEN, J., BLACK, L., *et al* (1990) Turn it sround: short term management of aggression and anger. *Journal of Psychosocial Nursing*, **28**, 6–12.

TURNER, J. (1984*a*) Preface. V*iolence in the Medical Care Setting: A Survival Guide* (ed. J. Turner). Colorado: Aspen.

—— (1984*b*) Hostage incidents in health care settings. In *Violence in the Medical Care Setting: A Survival Guide* (ed. J. Turner). Colorado: Aspen.

—— (1984*c*) Role of the ED nurse in health-care based hostage incidents. *Journal of Emergency Nursing*, **10**, 190–193.

WENK, E., ROBINSON, J. O. & SMITH, G. W. (1972) Can violence be prevented? *Violence and Delinquency*, **18**, 393–394.

WHITMAN, R. M., ARMAS, B. B. & DENT, O. B. (1976) Assaults on the therapist. *American Journal of Psychiatry*, **133**, 426–429.

WONDRAK, R. (1989) Dealing with verbal abuse. *Nurse Education Today*, **9**, 276–280.

5   The medical management of violence

MARGARET C. ORR and JOHN H. MORGAN

As part of the multidisciplinary team the psychiatrist plays a role in many aspects of the management of violence associated with mental disorder, but there are three areas where the medical/psychiatric contribution is essential: firstly in the application of mental health legislation; secondly in the prescribing of medication; and lastly in the authorisation of the use of seclusion in accordance with the *Code of Practice*. This chapter seeks to summarise these three topics in the medical management of violence. It concludes with a brief outline of some of the facilities in the United Kingdom which cater for the mentally ill who may be violent.

The application of the Mental Health Acts

The MHA 1983 refers to the Mental Health Act 1983, and applies to England and Wales. MH(S)A 1984 refers to the Mental Health (Scotland) Act 1984, and applies to Scotland. Summaries of the provisions of these Acts are given in Appendices 1–4 of the chapter.

The acute episode

In the Mental Health Acts three questions are addressed before a person may be detained:

(a) Is mental disorder present or suspected?
(b) Is the person's health at risk or is he/she a danger to himself/herself or others? (This is explicit only in MHA 1983.)
(c) What is the least level of security under which the person is likely to obtain the correct assessment and/or treatment?

These three basic precepts hold whenever the Mental Health Acts are applied and are as true for the police constable about to arrest the person under the terms of section 136 (MHA 1983) or 118 (MH(S)A 1984) as for the consultant psychiatrist who recommends detention under section 3 (MHA 1983) or 18 (MH(S)A 1984) – the most restrictive sections available to the psychiatrist.

The application of the Mental Health Acts in the community

Police detention – section 136 MHA 1983 and section 118 MH(S)A 1984

Under section 136 and 118, if a constable finds, in a place to which the public have access, a person who appears to be suffering from mental disorder and to be in immediate need of care or control, the constable may, if he/she thinks it necessary to do so in the interests of that person or for the protection of other persons, remove that person to a place of safety.

Detention is for a maximum of 72 hours and ends at time of medical and social work assessment. Examination is made as soon as possible by a registered medical practitioner and approved social worker.

Courts would interpret a public place as defined by common law to mean a place to which the public have access at the relevant time. Difficulties have arisen in considering places such as railway terminals, theatres, football stadiums and private blocks of flats.

Once in the 'place of safety', as defined in section 135 of MHA 1983, police are free to go, as the power to detain may be passed over to the managers of that establishment. However, a hospital is not legally obliged to admit the patient and indeed this section should definitely not be used as a substitute for an emergency admission under the section described below. The provision of both a registered medical practitioner and a social worker ensures an emergency section 24 MH(S)A 1984 can be immediately instigated if the need arises.

Section 135 defines the place of safety as residential accommodation (Part III), a hospital defined by Act, a mental nursing home or residential home for mentally disordered people or any other suitable place the occupier of which is willing to receive the patient temporarily. Only in exceptional circumstances can a police station be used, although in practice this depends on local arrangements made between the psychiatric services and the local police. If a hospital is used the patient cannot be moved from there to another hospital for treatment unless another part of the Act is used (e.g. section 24).

The police are generally right in their suspicions of mental disorder being present and in most cases where section 136 in England and Wales is used the assessing psychiatrist later confirms the presence of illness (Bean *et al*, 1990, 1991).

The Scottish Act does not define an assessment by a social worker but does state that the police constable should inform the responsible person living with the patient and the nearest relative if not one and the same.

Emergency admissions – section 4 in England and Wales, section 24 in Scotland

In both Mental Health Acts provision is made for emergency admission of a patient for assessment of the suspected mental disorder. The sections should only be used where urgency is paramount and not to do so would cause risk to the patient or others.

Applications of the Act to in-patients

In-patients are defined as those who have accepted an offer of a bed by appearing on a ward and cooperating with admission. It does not apply to out-patients or day-hospital patients.

Nurses' 'holding' powers – section 5(4) MHA 1983, section 25 MH(S)A 1984

In England and Wales if a first-level nurse considers an informal in-patient to be suffering from a mental disorder to the degree which endangers his/her health or safety or the safety of others, that patient should be restrained from leaving the hospital if he/she tries to do so. The patient may be stopped from leaving for up to six hours, during which time the registered medical practitioner in charge of the case must attend to decide whether an emergency order should be instigated under section 5(2). The doctor may have only one nominated deputy.

In Scotland nursing staff have a similar responsibility under section 25(2), but they have only two hours in which to summon medical attendance; the emergency procedure is the same as in section 24. In both Acts the nurse must record that the patient is suffering from mental disorder, that the patient has been detained, and the time for which the patient was first detained. This report has then to be taken to the hospital managers as soon as possible and in Scotland the managers must send a copy to the Mental Welfare Commission within 14 days.

Doctors' 'holding' powers

In the English Act a patient detained by nurses' holding powers may be made subject to detention under section 5(2) of the Act for 72 hours if the medical practitioner in charge of the patient's treatment makes a recommendation to the hospital managers. This power cannot be used to extend an emergency section 4 but is to allow a review of the patient in hospital and consideration of instigation of section 2 or 3 or discharge by the responsible medical officer.

Patients in accident and emergency departments, out-patient clinics or day hospitals

Under common law it is the right of any private individual to detain, in a situation of necessity, a person of unsound mind who is a danger to himself/herself or others (*Times*, 1988). The detention should, of course, be for as short a time as possible to allow the emergency procedures to operate. The common-law doctrine of necessity might also allow a short-acting sedative to be administered to the patient if communication is impossible. This is the reasoning behind administration of medication against the will in prisons, where the Mental Health Acts do not apply. It must only be used as a last resort and good practice should operate at all times.

Section 2 (MHA 1983) and section 26 (MH(S)A 1984)

Section 2 should be used for assessment when it seems likely that treatment in hospital will follow. The curtailment of liberty cannot be used simply to observe how someone behaves. It should not be forgotten that this section and section 3 are to be used also in cases where it is the patient's health (mental and physical) which is seriously at risk.

Although section 26 is of the same duration as the English section 2 (*vis* 28 days), it does not make any comment about separating assessment and treatment but simply states admission to hospital. It also only requires one medical recommendation.

In neither Act may the sections be renewed or an emergency section added. The medical team must make up their minds in the 28 days available whether the patient requires prolonged detention under sections 3 (England and Wales) or 18 (Scotland), or whether they will become informal.

Section 3 (MHA 1983) and section 18 (MH(S)A 1984)

Section 3 is used where the diagnosis is clear and agreed by the two recommending doctors, the need for treatment has been demonstrated and, since the 1983 Act, in cases of psychopathically disordered patients, that the treatment is liable to prevent deterioration or alleviate distress.

Renewal of detention under section 3 may be granted only if the registered medical practitioner certifies either that treatment is likely to alleviate or prevent deterioration or that the patient could not look after himself/herself in the community without serious exploitation or could not cope generally. This rule applies to mental illness, mental impairment and psychopathic disorder.

In Scotland, section 18 may be applied by a mental health officer or nearest relative who in each case has seen the patient within the 14 preceding days. (In England, two medical recommendations made within five days of each other must also be provided.) Application to the hospital managers must be approved by the sheriff within seven days and the section reviewed within two months. It can be renewed after six months, thereater annually as in England.

Rights of appeal

Mental Health Act 1983 – England and Wales

The patient may appeal to have a mental health review tribunal if detained under section 2 and the patient or the nearest relative may apply for a mental health review tribunal under section 3. The registered medical practitioner in charge of treatment of a patient admitted informally to hospital may delegate powers under section 5(2) to one (but only one) other doctor. Hospital managers are obliged to arrange mental health review tribunals for patients on section 3 every three years and the patient has the right to request a mental health review tribunal each year. Section 2 should be used where there is doubt about the actual diagnosis and it is felt the patient requires admission to clarify this and to provide a course of treatment, after which it is hoped the patient will either decide to continue with treatment voluntarily or be discharged. The patient may require to have the section 2 order converted to a section 3 order.

Mental Health (Scotland) Act 1984 – Scotland

In Scotland the Mental Welfare Commission and the sheriff carry out many of the functions which in England are carried out by the mental health review tribunals and the hospital advisory committees.

With emergency detentions hospital managers must inform the Mental Welfare Commission as soon as possible (as well as the nearest relative and any reliable person living with the patient if not the same person). Where nurses' holding powers have been used, a copy of the report is made to the hospital managers as soon as possible after the event. This should be sent to the Mental Welfare Commission within 14 days of the manager receiving it. Patients detained under the short-term section 26 (28 days) must have their case notified to the Mental Welfare Commission not later than seven days after detention. They have the right to appeal to the sheriff for release, as have all detained patients.

For those admitted under the provisions described in sections 18–23 the sheriff must approve the application with the medical recommendations and the patient is then admitted within seven days of that approval. The Mental Welfare Commission and the local authority for the area in which the hospital is situated must then be informed within seven days of the actual admission. The Mental Welfare Commission regularly visit hospitals in which detained patients are resident. They enquire into the conditions and may request interviews with the detained patients and any other patients in the hospital. They must see all section 18 patients annually and if they decide a patient should be discharged they make recommendations to the Secretary of State. They may inspect the patient's medical records and interview the patient's psychiatrist, but there is no formal tribunal system as in England.

Consent to treatment (Part IV MHA 1983 and Part X MH(S)A 1984)

The most recent Mental Health Acts attempted to clarify the situation where a responsible medical officer may treat a detained patient without his/her consent and these are described in Part IV of the English and Welsh Act and Part X of the Scottish Act. Another helpful explanation is given in Chapter 16 of the *Code of Practice*, Mental Health Act 1983.

This part of the Act does not apply to those detained on emergency orders, those detained by a nurse's holding power or "found in a public place" (136 and 118), or a conditionally discharged restricted patient (and also those detained under section 378 of the Criminal

Procedure Scotland Act 1975). These patients can be treated only under common law. Patients subject to guardianship and informal patients are not "liable to be detained", thus Part IV does not apply. However, those who have been granted leave of absence (under section 17 of the MHA 1983, or section 27 of the MH(S)A 1984) do come under the consent-to-treatment rules, and general practitioners must be informed of the consent forms completed by the original responsible medical officer or supervising psychiatrist as he/she will have to abide by them.

There is a 'three-month rule' which allows a responsible medical officer to treat a detained patient for three months from the first date on which he/she received one dose of medication. However, in this time it is important that the responsible medical officer seeks the patient's consent and finds a treatment acceptable to both so that the responsible medical officer may complete form 38, "Consent to Treatment" (MHA 1983) or form 9 (MH(S)A 1984). After three months the responsible medical officer must either confirm the patient is continuing to agree to the medication or have obtained the second-opinion appointed doctor (SOAD) from the Mental Health Act Commission – form 39 (MHA 1983) or form 10 (MH(S)A 1984).

Emergency treatment

In an emergency, section 62 (MHA 1983) or section 102 (MH(S)A 1984) may be used:

(a) to save a patient's life
(b) to prevent a serious deterioration (treatment must not be irreversible)
(c) to alleviate serious suffering (treatment must not be irreversible)
(d) to prevent violence to himself/herself or others (treatment must not be irreversible or hazardous).

Sections 62(2) and 102(2) allow for a course of treatment such as electroconvulsive therapy to be continued after withdrawal of consent if serious suffering would result to the patient, but the responsible medical officer must be attempting to comply with obtaining a second-opinion doctor. Hospital managers must supply a suitable form for recording emergency treatment under this provision and keep a register of the number of times the section is used. In England and Wales the hospital managers are informed and in Scotland the Mental Welfare Commission must be informed within seven days.

Consent to treatment means exploring with the patient not only the likely benefits and side-effects of the treatment but also what might happen if the patient did not have the treatment. This means a fine line being drawn between coercion and persuasion to give something which the doctor believes is necessary for the patient's health. The doctor has a duty of treatment and the patient a right to information and to give true informed consent.

Patients concerned in criminal proceedings or who are under sentence – the application of Part III of MHA 1983 and Part VI of MH(S)A 1984 and the Criminal Procedures Insanity Act

These sections relate to hospital orders imposed by courts and transfer of prisoners from prison to hospital. Those sections relating to offender patients are available only through the courts or at the direction of the Secretary of State and are thus outside the direct control of the health professional, although the sections cannot be implemented without the recommendations of medical professionals. Part III MHA 1983 and Part VI MH(S)A 1984 attempt to ensure that a mentally disordered person who commits an offence or is suspected of committing an offence will receive the proper assessment and treatment. Also those offenders who have developed mental disorder while serving a sentence are able to be transferred from prison to hospital if they are considered to be in need of treatment by the prison health staff and the visiting psychiatrists. (Details are contained in Appendixes III and IV.)

Guardianship

Provision for this has been made in both Acts (section 37 MHA 1983 and section 36 MH(S)A 1984) but whether through lack of knowledge in their use, lack of need or lack of power of the guardian, the facility is infrequently used. They were considered by the Butler committee to be a "useful form of control of some mentally disordered offenders who do not require hospital treatment, particularly suited to the needs of the subnormal offenders who require help in managing their affairs" (Home Office and Department of Health and Social Security, 1975, para. 15.8).

In Scotland it is specified that the person must be at least 16-years-old, suffering from a mental disorder which justifies admission into guardianship (medical grounds) and that it is in the interests of the welfare of the person that he/she be so admitted (welfare grounds). The person has to have committed an offence which could result in imprisonment if convicted; the guardian must be willing to accept the person into guardianship (usually social services); the person must have a mental disorder agreed by both recommending doctors (one of whom is approved) and no other sentence (e.g. probation order) must be passed. The advantage over a probation order is that the person need not agree to the guardianship but the disadvantage over the hospital order is that there is no authorisation for even three months of psychiatric treatment against the patient's wishes.

The guardian can decide where the patient lives, ensure the patient attends for medical treatment, work, education or training and insist that supervisors, including psychiatrists, have access to the patient. The guardian must provide regular reports and information to the social work department, notifying them of any change of address or general practitioner and any absences from residence or work. The guardian cannot however sign on behalf of the patient for any treatment carried out, financial transactions, or administer corporal punishment (*in loco parentis*). The latter is a statutory criminal offence in Scotland, which must be reported by the court to the Mental Welfare Commission.

The order may be discharged by the responsible medical officer, the social work department, the Mental Welfare Commission (in Scotland), the nearest relative or the sheriff (also in Scotland). The nearest relative must give not less than 14 days' notice in writing to the local authority concerned and may be overruled by the responsible medical officer or social services.

The prescribing of medication

The acute incident

Successful management of an acute act of violence aims at shortening the episode and averting further acts, reducing morbidity/disability to the victim and preventing further patient, family or staff distress. The least restrictive method of dealing with a dangerous situation is to be fostered. The practical management is detailed in Chapter 4. The aim of medication is to gain control of the situation to allow other intervention to be effective.

Medication should not be automatically used in a violent episode, as no drug is without hazard. Even if the decision to medicate has been taken, this should be reviewed regularly as response to treatment occurs.

The following approach is useful:

(a) Take a history. This is usually difficult and observers (staff or relatives) will be useful. From the history look out for:

(i)   indicators of a physical cause (e.g. a sudden onset – hours rather than days – in someone with no history of psychiatric disorder is suggestive of an organic condition)

(ii)   sudden onset in someone with a history of psychiatric disorder but no history of violence also indicates the need for investigation of organic cause

(iii)   recurrence of violence in a psychiatric patient with a history of violence but no obvious precipitant such as change in medication should also raises doubts, and a physical cause should be excluded

(iv)   one should also consider illegal drug use, alcohol abuse or head injury; even trivial head trauma may cause a chronic subdural haematoma in the alcoholic or elderly person, and a sudden change in behaviour may be the first indication (those on anticoagulants are also at risk of subdural bleeding after minor trauma).

(b) Do a mental state examination. This is rarely complete as the patient is often inaccessible owing to rage, fear or thought disorder, although in some cases the very act of violence has an expunging effect and calm may follow at least temporarily. Look for any sign of disorientation, impaired or fluctuating level of consciousness. Visual hallucinations or sensory illusions increase the likelihood of an organic cause. The disorganised thinking of the acute schizophrenic or manic patient may mimic confusion, but a fluctuation in level of attention is strongly suggestive of an organic state.

(c) Make a full physical examination. While a patient is lying on a floor being restrained by five people this is a daunting task, but a few basic recordings provide clues to diagnosis and treatment. The patient should be told when and where you are going to touch him/her. Even the most belligerent psychotic person can often understand and it may lessen the fear to hear a friendly voice. The precepts of examination by looking, smelling and listening before touching should be encouraged. Look for:

(i)   needle marks, bruises or ligature marks on the arms suggestive of drug abuse

(ii)   the smell of alcohol or acetone will also provide clues as to alcoholic intoxication, diabetes or neglect

(iii)   any elevation of temperature in a confused and violent person suggests that the disturbance may be secondary to infection elsewhere; the possibility of neuroleptic malignant syndrome should be borne in mind in those already medicated

(iv) pulse and respiration abnormalities can suggest heart failure, decreased cerebral blood flow, salicylate poisoning, and so on

(v) the head should be examined as closely as possible by observation and touch and particular attention paid to the cranial nerves. At the very least, pupil reaction should be attempted.

This assessment should lead to some kind of formulation or diagnosis which will lead to appropriate treatment or referral.

Psychiatric diagnoses associated with violence

The most common psychiatrically disordered violent patient presenting at casualty is young, male and schizophrenic (Mullen, 1988). There may be an overlap not only with personality disorder but also with substance or alcohol abuse, but it has been shown consistently that the level of violence in schizophrenic patients is higher than in other diagnostic groups and the population at large. This has been confirmed in the major prison study by Taylor & Gunn (1984; Taylor, 1985), and in a ten-year study in West Germany the risk of violent offending in schizophrenics was found to be 0.05%, twice that in the population generally. These findings have been confirmed by Fottrell *et al* (1978). However, it also needs to be said that most young male schizophrenics are not violent.

The next most common mental illness presenting with violence in accident and emergency is mania or hypomania where there is marked agitation, irritability and anger at being frustrated in their expansive desires. The other pole of affective disorder, the depressive, can also be violent. For example, someone who has attempted suicide and is having the wounds stitched, may suddenly see no way out of the world and become homicidal. Such cases are however rare.

The personality-disordered patient is the third most likely to be violent towards self or others. Their impulsivity and lack of concern for the effect on others mean they can be especially dangerous.

The indication for medication

A patient who remains distressed and struggling, shouting and abusive with no sign of stopping some time after the original incident is in danger of becoming exhausted and is in a most degrading situation which can do little for long-term needs or relationships with staff. It is impossible to be prescriptive on the time to allow before administering drugs, as each unit has its own tolerance for such events. However, the wellbeing of the patient should be a priority. Some would advise giving medication before attempting to move the patient, as it is certainly during the moving of disturbed patients that further violent incidents often occur (Tupin, 1983). It may be difficult, however, to provide sufficient steadying of the patient in a clear enough light to allow parenteral medication to be administered. In the best scenario, the patient is persuaded to relax and accept oral medication sitting on the floor and then helped to a nearby chair to allow continued counselling with a known nurse or doctor. Where this is not possible it is worthwhile improving visibility to the area by bringing in extra light and essential to hold the patient as still as possible and explain what is going to happen.

Each clinical team has its own favoured drug regimen but it must be stated that no psychotropic medication is without its side-effects, and interactions with other drugs must be considered. The risk of damage to the patient (up to and including death) has to be weighed against the risk of leaving him/her untreated.

Appropriate drugs

A fast-acting drug with a short duration of action to allow re-assessment of the situation is to be preferred. Few side-effects, reliable absorption by a range of routes and low irritability on injection are all features to be looked for. The perfect drug has yet to be found, although improvements are developing yearly. Modern treatment after an acutely violent incident relies on two main groups of drugs or a combination of both. They are the antipsychotics/neuroleptics and the benzodiazepines.

Antipsychotics/neuroleptics are a group of drugs so called because of their action on specific systems in the central nervous system. In the acute situation they are used for their tranquillising effect. The antipsychotics haloperidol and droperidol (both belonging to the butyrophenone group) have similar properties to the phenothiazines (chlorpromazine) but have less effect on the cardiovascular system, can be given intravenously or intramuscularly, have rapid onset (droperidol intravenously or intramuscularly works within five to ten minutes) and they are less anticholinergic. However, they must still be used with caution and each case judged on its own needs regarding size of patient, degree of disturbance, responsiveness of tissues and concentration of drug at site of action, and it is thus not possible to give a maximum correct dosage. These drugs can cause serious side-effects of dystonia, akathisia (extreme restlessness, particularly in the legs) and at least one case of cardiac arrest following intravenous use has been described (Huyse *et al*, 1988). A full description of the common neuroleptics used in this situation is contained in Appendix 5.

Considerations when using antipsychotics in the acute situation

Acute dystonia. This severe distressing muscular reaction should be treated with immediate procyclidine hydrochloride (10 mg intramuscularly or 5 mg intravenously).

Epilepsy. The fit threshold for epileptic patients is reduced by neuroleptics and thought should be given to increasing the level of anticonvulsant being taken (if any).

Neuroleptic malignant syndrome. This may occur with neuroleptics and should be recognised and treated early by withdrawing the offending drug. Symptoms/signs are increased temperature and muscle tone, high blood pressure and rapid pulse, and disordered mental state, from delirium to coma. If suspected, intramuscular injections should be avoided and blood sent for analysis of white cell count and creatinine phosphokinase levels, which will be raised. This is a medical emergency and will require admission to a medical intensive-care unit.

Benzodiazepines

Benzodiazepines can be useful in violent patients where antipsychotics are not recommended (e.g. where fitting has occurred, where alcohol is complicating the picture and where severe dystonia has occurred in the past with neuroleptics). The commonest of the group to be used in an emergency are diazepam and lorazepam. The latter can be useful where liver damage is present, as it is not metabolised by the liver. All benzodiazepines can cause confusion, oversedation and ataxia, particularly in the elderly. They have been used recently in combination with neuroleptics in what is known as rapid tranquillisation.

Rapid tranquillisation

This term is defined by Dubin (1988) as a circumscribed procedure of giving varying amounts of antipsychotic medication over brief intervals (30–60 minutes) to control agitated, threatening and potentially destructive patients, with most patients responding in one to four hours.

The preferred route for rapid tranquillisation has been intramuscular because of rapid absorption and greater bio-availability of the drug. A survey by Pilowsky *et al* (1992) showed all three routes of administration being used as well as a wide range of dosages of six different drugs – diazepam, haloperidol, droperidol, chlorpromazine, lorazepam and paraldehyde. In this survey, rapid tranquillisation was used as a last resort and it was suggested that more interest be paid to the group of patients who have severe illness and physically aggressive behaviour, as they require vigorous treatment before they harm themselves or others.

It would seem that the way forward in the pharmacological management of the acutely violent patient is to give a small dose of neuroleptics with or without adjuvant benzodiazepine and to repeat the injection if necessary according to patient need. However, the alternative action of zuclopenthixol acetate (Acuphase) may become the preference.

The repeatedly violent patient

The management of the repetitively violent person in a psychiatric hospital requires a multidisciplinary approach. Recognition of cycles of violence, prevention and the role of the management and environment are detailed elsewhere. It is essential that a full multidisciplinary assessment explores all treatment options in order to alleviate a patient's need to be violent. This will include observation, interview and trial of all therapeutic options, including psychotherapy – both cognitive, behavioural and dynamic. However, the patient's underlying mental disorder may be such that he/she is unamenable to any change in outlook or cognition. By noting the behaviour patterns and if possible performing an analysis of the behaviour, the psychiatrist may provide the appropriate medication to prevent the violence recurring. As with the acutely violent person, diagnosis comes before medication.

Organic causes

Dementia. The various types of organic dementia can all present with aggressive behaviour or violence, depending on the affected area of the brain. Where the frontal lobes are incorporated the irritability, fatuousness and sexual disinhibition may be a great problem and the violence needs to be contained by a structured environment and treatment programme. Dementing old people can be repetitively violent but rarely organised enough to kill. If they are inadequately supervised, however, and have access to other frail elderly people, they can occasionally kill their fellow residents. Strict observation and awareness of likely precipitants is essential in dealing with violence in the elderly and dementing.

Epilepsy. A survey of British epileptic prisoners did not reveal an association between temporal lobe epilepsy and violence (Dubin, 1988). Nevertheless, there are a few patients with epilepsy who end up in special hospitals because of their violence either pre- or postictally. It has to be stressed however that all of these are people with the additional diagnosis of schizophrenia superimposed on epilepsy.

Encephalitis. In one special hospital there has recently been a case of continuous serious violence in a patient with chronic brainstem encephalitis undiagnosed until post-mortem. These are rare cases but show among other things that where persistent violence is unamenable to medication, psychology and nursing, there may be additional factors of organic disease or serious personality disorders influencing presentation.

Functional causes related to psychosis

Delusions. The analysis of a disturbed incident may allow the multidisciplinary team to see repeating misidentifications. Where it turns out that a misinterpretation is founded upon a paranoid delusion in the case of a patient with a schizophrenic illness, the effect of medication will be a major issue. Any recent change in amount or combination of medication may be significant.

Hallucinations. There has been considerable interest in the role of hallucinations – particularly command hallucinations (i.e. those which order, ask or tell) – in the committing of violent acts. The underlying psychosis must be treated by oral or depot neuroleptics. It is part of the psychiatrist's role to be able to differentiate the true command hallucination from the common statements which are used to explain violence: "Something made me/told me/forced me to do it," "I couldn't help myself. Something came over me," or "I could hear her voice telling me to do it". Once again the symptom has to be placed in the context of observed behaviour and other symptoms of the schizophrenic illness.

Medication

If psychotic symptoms are an important influence, the patient will require antipsychotic medication. Patients should receive adequate regular medication to control symptoms using whichever depot or oral antipsychotic agent is most suited to the patient's needs, as it has been suggested that 'under-treatment' of the psychosis is one of the main factors in repetitive violence. No antipsychotic is without side-effects and hazards but most patients benefit from their use.

Depot injections are neuroleptic drugs which release the drug slowly into the circulation, allowing a patient to receive medication infrequently and often reducing side-effects.

The newer oral antipsychotic agents such as clozapine or risperidone have already shown dramatic effects on the aggressive behaviour of hospital patients, roughly a third of cases having symptoms relieved, a third being improved and a third no worse. Lack of compliance and difficulties in gaining the cooperation of the disturbed patient to have the necessary weekly blood tests for at least the first 18 weeks of treatment remain obstacles, but where all other depot antipsychotic medications have been tried both within and above the limits set in the *British National Formulary*, there is a place to try clozapine. The toxicity of the drug, with the possibility of neutropenia and fatal agranulocytosis and other serious side-effects (myocarditis, delusions and, rarely, circulatory collapse), makes the drug hazardous but the benefits can be significant. Risperidone, without the same haematological affects, shows promise but both drugs are new and expensive.

Mood disorders

Depressive symptoms. Patients may remain persistently violent to others as a result of continuing feelings of hopelessness, needing to rid themselves of their supposed tormentors or project their own bad feelings on to others. Clues to the underlying depressive component may come from features such as:

(a) irritability in mornings with worsening of attacks
(b) cutting themselves or head banging when prevented from hitting others
(c) attacking others at meal times when even the sight of food arouses their awareness of depression
(d) disturbance and shouting back at derogatory voices.

It is easier to identify causes of the irritability and violence if patients are expressing their thoughts, looking unhappy and have a history of depression, but it is occasionally the schizophrenic patient who has been stabilised on medication only to become repetitively violent who is masking superimposed depression. It is worth undertaking a trial of antidepressant with or without lithium to treat such cases but care must be taken with drug interaction and potentiation. The role of anniversaries in repetitive violence should be acknowledged.

Hypomania and violence. Elevation of mood may also give rise to repetitive violence. Hypomania in the manic–depressive patient or a manic phase in a schizoaffective disorder may result in violence.

In cases of chronic hypomania with disinhibition, irritability and repeated acts of violence where treatment has only achieved short periods of relative stability, attention should be given to complicating factors of additional physical disorders (e.g. hyperthyroidism, infection, metabolic disorders) and social factors which contribute to the perpetuation of the 'illness mode' (e.g. loss of family and social isolation).

Side-effects of medication

Drugs given for the treatment of psychosis may contribute to violence. For example akathisia can make the patient so uncomfortably restless that he/she will strike out.

Rationale of pharmacological management

Attempts have been made to rationalise the pharmacological management of violence based on anatomical, neurophysiological and neurobiochemical research in animals and human studies (Connoly, 1985). Three types of aggressive behaviour are suggested: predatory; defensive; and frustration. These have been linked with specific areas of the brain and three neurotransmitters: gamma-aminobutyric acid (GABA); noradrenaline (in the locus coeruleus) and serotonin (in the Raphé nucleus). It is also suggested that there is a neurophysiological basis for aggression. Animal studies have shown that subictal stimulation (i.e. electrical stimulation which does not produce a fit), when administered to certain areas of the brain, can reduce aggressive behaviour and fits. Human studies have indicated higher levels of electroencephalographic (EEG) abnormalities in aggressive offenders and aggressive men.

The interest in the three neurotransmitter systems and their role in aggressive behaviour lies in the fact that they may indicate a more rational way to treat violence. The schizophrenic person might require an ongoing smaller dose of depot with adjuvant medication to relieve violent episodes.

The GABA system. When activated this system lowers aggression in animals. Benzodiazepines are able to activate GABA receptors. Their limitations/side-effects however are that they are rapidly tolerated and have considerable withdrawal difficulties. It is thus essential to limit their use to short courses and not to repeat the course quickly. Previous reports of paradoxical rage being released when benzodiazepines are used (Bond & Lader, 1979) have not been strongly supported by clinical data (Sheard, 1984). Although there have been isolated reports of episodes of paradoxical rage in normal and aggressive subjects, there has been a suggestion that when given to caged animals, benzodiazepines increase their likelihood to have explosive outbursts. This may have relevance when considering the use of benzodiazepines in institutions where the patients have inadequate personal space.

The noradrenergic system. This system is activated in defensive or reactive aggression where avoidance of pain, either physical or emotional, is the driving force. However, it generally inhibits predatory aggressive behaviour where the aim is to achieve a reward. Part of the mode of action of tricyclic antidepressants (such as imipramine and amitriptyline) is to increase noradrenergic activity, while beta-blockers (such as propranolol) decrease activity. It is suggested that propranolol (40 mg twice or three times daily) may reduce aggression, particularly in brain injured (Sorgi *et al*, 1986) and/or refractory schizophrenic subjects (Tupin, 1978). Its mode of action appears to be peripheral as well as central, providing symptomatic relief of tension. It takes some days to reach effective control, however, so its place lies in the long-term management of violence. One of the actions of lithium is to decrease noradrenergic activity and, in addition to its usual mood-stabilising action, it has also been found to have an inhibitory effect on aggression in both animals and man (Craft *et al*, 1987). This effect has been shown in chronic psychotic, mentally impaired and personality-disordered patients (Greenberg *et al*, 1976). It is suggested that the common link in the group is the hair-trigger temper, a lack of reflection before the response, and an inability to modulate the response.

The serotonergic system. Like the GABA system, this neurotransmitter system appears to be inhibitory for aggression. Lowering its production would be likely to increase aggression and raising its production would decrease aggression. In the rat both predatory and defensive aggressive behaviour is increased by restricting the dietary intake of tryptophan, the biological precursor of serotonin. Human studies have corroborated the evidence that tryptophan metabolism is involved in aggression. In a population of hyperactive children aggressive behaviour was linked to low levels of serotonin and serotonin-like compounds (Klegman & Goldberg, 1975). Others have reported a decrease in aggression in a group of schizophrenic patients treated with 4–8 g tryptophan per day.

Neurophysiological aspects of violence and its treatment. There has long been an association between epilepsy and aggression, though at times it has possibly been exaggerated (Gunn & Brown, 1971; Turks & Dermen, 1977). The periodicity of aggressive behaviour in epilepsy is well known (epileptic equivalents, epileptoid phenomena, epileptic psychoses). The outbursts were particularly evident in the days before the anticonvulsant phenytoin was introduced. The disinhibitory effect of phenobarbitone and other early anticonvulsants may have contributed, but it is still suspected that subclinical seizure activity may be responsible for some of the aggressive behaviour exhibited by some epileptic people. Subcortical epileptic discharges have been found in some schizophrenic patients who were in remission and in cases where there is an association between temporal-lobe spiking as recorded on EEG and violent behaviour. This is the rationale behind using carbamazepine, an anticonvulsant useful in all types of epilepsy apart from absence seizures and in prophylaxis of manic–depressive episodes. It is structurally related to the tricyclic antidepressants. An open study by Turks & Dermen (1977) found it to be successful with episodic dyscontrol patients and it has been used as an adjunct to control excited psychotics. However, controlled studies have been disappointing (Sheard, 1984). Despite this some continue to use it for uncontrolled outbursts of rage.

Seclusion in the management of violence

The history of seclusion

The concept of restraining or isolating patients in psychological distress is not a new one. Writers in the first and second centuries AD refer to the practice of chaining and binding those unresponsive to the treatments of the times (Jones, 1988). In the 19th century, following the abandonment of physical restraint in asylums, enforced isolation was viewed as a humane alternative to shackles as long as it was conducted without negative motivations such as anger, contempt, neglect or punishment (Kalogjera *et al*, 1989).

Seclusion practices have endured the revolution in psychiatry created by the concept of a therapeutic milieu and the discovery of the antipsychotics in the 1950s (Jones, 1988). There is general acceptance that their use is confined to the most difficult of presenting problems, usually involving high levels of verbal or physical aggression on the part of a patient. A broad theoretical base justifying the use of seclusion was proposed by Gutheil (1978). Gutheil's 'theory of seclusion' was based on three principles: safety in the form of containment, isolation, and reduction in sensory stimulation.

Containment refers to the restriction of the patient's movements, in order to prevent harm to self or others and to protect the patient from the likely consequences of his/her actions. A psychoanalytic perspective sees the room in which the patient is isolated as a more effective and tangible set of boundaries than those provided by personal relationships (Hodgkinson, 1985).

Isolation is said to allow for the fact that a patient in distress has difficulties in establishing and interpreting personal relationships. Being placed in a small room provides an opportunity for the patient to master available space while sheltered from the distress caused by confused interpretations of dealings with others.

Reduction in sensory stimulation aims to reduce psychotic over-sensitivity or hyperaesthesia, which may contribute to behavioural disturbance. Seclusion is purported to offer a state of therapeutic monotony in the patient's environment.

Clinical value of seclusion

Gutheil's principles suggest a degree of clinical validity in the use of seclusion. Aside from it having the practical benefits of removing a challenging patient from the immediate environment, there is the suggestion that it is a specific treatment applied to ameliorate the disabilities exhibited by a patient in responding to experiences. There is a need to review the evidence for its effectiveness as a treatment and to examine any risks which might occur through its use.

It is suggested that seclusion is an extension of the therapeutic relationship, within which the person's controls are maintained. Performance indicators arising from this suggestion examine the relationship between patients and staff subsequent to seclusion being used, the effects on the target behaviour towards which seclusion is directed, and a service-user perspective on the experience of seclusion with regard to its acceptability as a practice and its effects on the individual's wellbeing.

Seclusion and staff–patient relationships

Soliday (1985) surveyed staff and patient attitudes to seclusion in a psychiatric hospital in Kansas; 86 patients and 37 staff (representing return rates of 59% and 66% respectively) completed questionnaires. All were placed across three wards where 'seclusion' involved the placement of the patient in a "regular sleeping room that has no furniture except for a mattress and a blanket. A nursing staff member checks the status of a secluded patient every 15 minutes and a physician checks the person every three hours."

The patient group, both those who had been secluded (65%) and those who had not, showed a more negative attitude to seclusion than did the staff. In terms of its effect on staff–patient relationships, seclusion was said by 45% of patients to lead to distrust of staff. Only

16% of staff felt this to be the case, the difference being statistically significant ($P = 0.001$). When staff and patients were asked whether seclusion made patients dislike staff, 54% of patients and 15% of staff responded in the affirmative.

Of the patient group, 16% felt that seclusion "usually" humiliated people, 35% felt that this was "always" the case; 22% said that seclusion was "usually", and 45% said it was "always" felt as punishment; 13% said that seclusion "usually" depressed people with 32% saying that this was always the case. In addition to the feelings of punishment, humiliation and depression, perceptual distortions, including seeing "beautiful lights", derealisation and hearing frightening sounds were reported. Thirty-six per cent of patients "sometimes" felt that harm may come to them in seclusion while 48% said that seclusion made people want to harm themselves. Seventy-six per cent of the patients responded with "sometimes", "usually" or "always" to the item suggesting that seclusion shows that staff care, while 87% said that seclusion made the ward safer at least "sometimes" and 69% said that it made those secluded feel safe at least "sometimes". Fifty-seven per cent said that seclusion "usually" helped people calm down. It seems that the patient respondents to the questionnaire perceived some benefits to themselves as individuals through the existence of the facility to seclude.

Soliday's work describes a widely varying set of responses on behalf of the patient group, some of whom indicate that seclusion is a humiliating and depressing experience which they perceive as punishment. A sizable minority felt that seclusion made patients distrust staff and a small majority said that it made patients dislike staff. In terms of the criterion of benefiting the staff–patient relationship, there is little to suggest that seclusion in this study was effective.

The positive aspects of seclusion indicated by the patients' responses have been challenged by Chamberlin (1985), who commented that:

> "patients and ex-patients commonly view seclusion as a form of torture. This is true not only of activists . . . ; most patients, when given the chance to speak in a supportive and non-punitive atmosphere, will speak negatively of their experience of seclusion."

Chamberlin raises the issue of the validity of the patient responses, alluding to a tendency for patients to "play the game". The 'game' involves acknowledging the therapeutic benefit of unpleasant treatment experiences in order to avoid their repetition and facilitate speedier discharge from hospital. Her view is that the patient responses might be contaminated by such tactics. A further criticism of the results presented by Soliday is the grouping together of patients who had been secluded and those who had not: this precludes any examination of the effects of seclusion on the people who are subject to its practice directly.

Chamberlin suggests a situation where patients distort their opinions in order to manipulate certain outcomes for themselves: thus there is the danger of seclusion introducing dishonesty into the staff–patient relationship, with potentially negative consequences. This, in conjunction with the aforementioned distrust and dislike of staff on the part of patients, raises serious doubts about the possibility of seclusion enhancing staff–patient relationships. Furthermore, the sense of punishment, humiliation and depression experienced by some patients because of its use implies that seclusion might be counter-therapeutic.

Seclusion and mental state

Other North American studies suggest that seclusion may have a negative effect on the patient's mental state (Plutchik *et al*, 1978; Wadeson & Carpenter, 1976; Binder & McCoy, 1983). Effects noted have included pleasurable visual hallucinations, unpleasant or terrifying delusions, depression, boredom, anger, disgust, confusion, helplessness and fear. These findings are difficult to interpret for two reasons. Firstly, a range of studies suggest a tendency to use seclusion predominantly for patients described as "disturbed and disruptive" (Plutchik *et al*, 1978; Soloff & Turner, 1981; Russel *et al*, 1985; Mattson & Sacks, 1978). This lack of precision may confuse clinical state with the environmental effect of the patient's behaviour. Such a term does not allow one to say whether the patient is being secluded because of a deterioration in mental state, behaviour or the ability of the staff to deal with either of these. Secondly, it is difficult to determine whether some of the symptoms or reactions experienced by patients in seclusion would not have occurred had their crisis been managed in another way.

To say that psychotic symptoms have occurred in seclusion does not mean to say that it has caused them. There is some evidence, however, which has linked the experience of solitary confinement in prisons with the emergence of psychiatric symptoms. Grassian (1983) presents evidence both from a clinical survey of North American prisoners subject to solitary confinement and from the literature of the late 19th and early 20th centuries. He suggests that some prisoners under particularly severe forms of solitary confinement develop perceptual changes (hyper-responsivity to external stimuli, perceptual distortions, hallucinations and derealisation experiences), acute anxiety attacks, cognitive impairments (confusion, partial amnesia, poor concentration), disturbances of thought content (upsetting violent revenge fantasies, ideas of reference and paranoia) and problems of impulse control (leading to violence both to self and property). The symptoms reported usually subsided within the first few hours after the termination of solitary confinement.

To generalise the findings from Grassian's sample to users of mental health services would not be valid – he describes reactions of offenders with unknown psychiatric histories to being locked in a room with only a small perspex window, with human contact only at mealtimes, for between eleven days and ten months. There is no information on the duration of solitary confinement before the onset of the experiences noted. Nonetheless, the emergence of disturbing symptoms in his sample, and the similarity of these to the experiences of patients in seclusion, presents as a caution in basing judgements about the need to continue seclusion episodes purely on the mental state of the patient. Where the patient has endured long periods of time away from human contact the possibility of seclusion contributing to any abnormal experiences or interpretations must be kept in mind.

Seclusion and behaviour change

A number of studies describe the wide range of conditions in which seclusion has been applied (Russell *et al*, 1986; Plutchik *et al*, 1978; Mattson & Sacks, 1978; Binder & McCoy, 1979; Soloff & Turner, 1981; Campbell *et al*, 1982). Categories of behaviour have emerged as follows: physical violence to staff; physical violence to patients; physical violence to property; threats of violence to staff; threats of violence to patients; disturbed and disruptive behaviour; self-injury. These seven categories are unlikely to be exhaustive. One survey (Campbell *et al*, 1982) cites a range of reasons recorded by nursing staff for the initiation of a seclusion episode which include absconding, arguing, verbal abuse of patients, stealing, lying and inciting other patients against staff. There are considerable difficulties of interpretation in reviewing the literature, with one author's disturbed and disruptive behaviour being another author's threatened violence.

The somewhat diffuse category of 'disturbed and disruptive behaviour' prompts a greater proportion of recorded seclusion episodes across the majority of studies. The survey by Campbell *et al* (1982) found that after seclusion 72% of patients were 'settled or apologetic' while 28% continued to be disruptive. The short-term effects on behaviour demonstrated in this study would suggest that seclusion is reasonably effective in managing an incident where risk is perceived by care staff. Russell *et al* (1986) suggest that it is not purely the behaviour displayed by a patient which would lead to seclusion. Mapping the frequency of initiation of seclusion across the working day, Russell and his colleagues found peaks around staff break times, when nurses were off the ward. Two attributions were made for this finding: firstly, that patient disturbance might be prompted by lower staff numbers; and secondly, that staff made the judgement to seclude earlier in the process of intervening in behavioural disturbance as a protective measure against escalation which might be difficult to contain with the available resources. This suggests that seclusion serves the function of containing staff anxiety as well as patient disturbance.

Longer-term effects on patient behaviour might well be difficult to demonstrate and there is little information on the effects of seclusion over time. Hodgkinson (1985) reports a personal communication from Sperlinger on the introduction of a seclusion policy on a long-stay ward for disturbed women. He found no decrease in the level of violent incidents recorded over six months compared with the preceding six months. Hodgkinson goes on to say that "no study has as yet measured objectively the same behaviours before and after seclusion, or has contrasted the use of seclusion with another procedure".

Seclusion is not specifically regulated by statute. It is however required that guidelines governing its use are in place. Such guidelines currently exist in the *Mental Health Act Code of Practice* (Department of Health, 1993).

Current definitions of seclusion and a framework for its use

Common themes within the definition of seclusion have included those of confinement, isolation, treatment, protection of others and protection of the client. The concept of seclusion as a treatment has found little acceptance over the decade since the publication of the Mental Health Act 1983. The *Code of Practice* (1993) states that, "Although it falls within the definition of medical treatment in the Mental Health Act (section 145), seclusion is not a treatment technique and should not feature as part of any treatment programme" (p. 77, para. 18.14). The *Code* deals with seclusion within the context of patients detained under the provisions of the MHA 1983. These patients might present particular management problems, including non-participation in treatment, prolonged verbal abuse/threatening behaviour, destructive behaviour, self-injury and physical attacks on others. If such difficulties occur with informal patients, treatment is initiated under common law. Jones (1988) quotes the Criminal Law

Act 1967 in the context of informal patients:

> "a person may use such force as is reasonable in the circumstances in the prevention of crime, or in effecting or assisting the lawful arrest of offenders or of suspected offenders unlawfully at large."

This provision allows members of staff to use reasonable force in the prevention of the commission of an assault or other offence. Reasonable steps are said to include the detention of a person against his/her will where a breach of the peace is threatened on either public or private property. While a breach of the peace is not necessarily an offence, the anticipation or reality of harm arising to either property or people empowers an individual to detain or seclude an informal patient for a limited period only. Should the need for prolonged detention become apparent then holding powers under the MHA 1983 should be sought.

The approach to management problems presented within the *Code* is hierarchical, one beginning with prevention, moving to restraint, both verbal and physical, using medication and finally placing the person in seclusion. Seclusion is defined by the *Code* both according to its nature and its purpose:

> "Seclusion is the supervised confinement of a patient alone in a room which may be locked for the protection of others from significant harm."

The *Code* stipulates that seclusion should be used as infrequently as possible for the least possible duration and only when all other methods have been employed. It should never be used where there is a risk of self-harm or suicide. These guidelines place responsibility on all carers, and have a strong emphasis on prevention. Prevention begins with the examination of all possible causes of problem behaviours within the person and in the environment, and the process of care delivery. The *Code* does not restrict itself to the need to prevent behaviours which prompt seclusion, however: it also prescribes actions consistent with good practice when this measure is undertaken. A more detailed examination of the prevention of violence is contained elsewhere.

Seclusion policies alone are unlikely to be enough to affect the frequency of its use. The availability of alternative management strategies appears to be the crucial factor. A systematic trial of an active prevention approach with adolescent in-patients in Wisconsin proved highly successful, with a 64% reduction in seclusion and restraint episodes over five months after its introduction. The number of patients requiring seclusion and restraint dropped by 39% over the same period (Kalogjera *et al*, 1989). The approach described may not be applicable to all patients, but does demonstrate the possible effect of active preventive management.

Seclusion policies may run in parallel to policies governing the administration of programmes based on learning theory, emphasising the difference between the concepts of behavioural containment and behavioural change (Gentry & Ostapiuk, 1988). Again, in this context, seclusion is a last resort which is not prescribed as a treatment but applied in order to interrupt a crisis and prevent further harm being done. This stands in contrast to the much misunderstood use of time-out procedures. These procedures are so classified because of their common aim of removing from the individual access to the positively reinforcing consequences of their maladaptive behaviour. The term is derived from the somewhat wordy description 'time out from positive reinforcement'. An analysis of a particular problem behaviour, perhaps loud wailing, may reveal that it is maintained by any form of attention from staff. In this case it might be that a three-pronged approach is taken. Firstly, staff may be instructed to give attention preferentially to other, more appropriate behaviours; secondly, staff may then ignore the wailing while, thirdly, the patient may receive training in more acceptable ways of communicating. In this package the time-out element is the ignoring of the wailing behaviour (i.e. the withholding of the usual reinforcer).

The picture emerging from the available literature is of seclusion as a means of removing a patient from the immediate environment, the main effect being the removal of opportunities to harm others or self and to allow for more settled behaviour to emerge. There is little evidence suggesting that seclusion contributes to long-term changes in behaviour.

There are suggestions that seclusion is used to the detriment of the relationship between staff and patients in some cases. Concerns have been raised about the potential for seclusion to have adverse effects on the patient's mental state, although at times part of the rationale for its use has been that it offers potential benefits in this regard. There are major difficulties in making sense of the literature, for the reasons given by Hodgkinson (1985), above. No evidence has been presented concerning the effect of seclusion on a specified set of behaviours, measured before and after the implementation of a seclusion regime, and seclusion is often implemented concurrently with emergency medication, thus preventing any identification of specific treatment effects.

The practice of seclusion is deservedly a controversial and an emotive one. The trend towards minimal restrictiveness within the care of the clients of psychiatric services has had a profound impact on service delivery throughout the spectrum of provision. Against this background the management of people in acute crisis still presents some of the most immediate challenges to direct-care staff in maintaining the ability of clients to make choices on their own behalf, especially where the person's state of mind leads to choices which threaten the safety of themselves and others. While some residential facilities operate non-seclusion policies there is a steady stream of referrals to more secure settings in which seclusion is resorted to.

Specialist facilities for the violent mentally disordered

There are three special hospitals in England (Broadmoor, Ashworth and Rampton) dealing with those of dangerous, violent or criminal propensities who require conditions of special security to conduct the treatment of their mental disorder. The State Hospital at Carstairs Junction provides this function for Scotland and Northern Ireland, while Dundrum supplies maximum-secure facilities in the Irish Republic. It would be expected that they would contain higher levels of violence towards fellow patients and staff than other facilities, and the two partial studies which have been reported upon have indeed reflected this (Larkin *et al*, 1988; Caldwell & Naismith, 1989). These studies also supported the work of Fottrell (1980) in general in-patient psychiatric hospitals by showing that a small proportion of the patients are responsible for most of the assaults. Factors such as ward culture, degree of activity (physical and mental), social mix of staff and patients, seasonal factors (higher levels in winter months), environmental factors and degree of mental disorder are all relevant and require a special training in management, with flexible and responsive approaches by staff of all disciplines. The hospitals provide a challenging environment for research, learning and development of techniques in the management of violence. The ability to respond to violent incidents with large numbers of staff drawn from other areas of the hospital has been seen as an important factor in retaining the size of the special hospitals, but this has now been challenged in recent reports (Bluglass, 1992). Once violence has erupted there is safety in numbers to prevent further damage to patient and staff alike, but increased knowledge of precipitants to violence is essential before embarking on potentially dangerous strategies.

The regional and subregional medium-secure units now in evidence throughout England and Wales exhibit considerably lower levels of violence. High staff:patient ratios and the ability to isolate

Summary points

- The Mental Health Act allows for the admission of patients against their will if: they are suffering from a treatable mental illness; they are likely to threaten themselves or others; they are refusing admission to hospital.
- There are essential differences between the Mental Health Acts in England & Wales (MHA 1983) and Scotland (MH(S)A 1984).
- Guidance on the use of the mental health act is contained in the *Code of Practice.*
- Medical treatment of violence should include a full multi-disciplinary assessment of all potential precipitants of violent behaviour.
- All medications are potentially hazardous.
- Medication should only be used after as full an assessment as possible has been undertaken and other treatments (e.g. 'talking down'; diversion /distraction) have failed.
- The dose should be titrated to the effectiveness of treatment and regularly reviewed.
- Seclusion should only be used as a last resort and never when the patient is suicidal.

incidents as well as patients who are less seriously repetitively violent and treatment resistant than those in the special hospitals may be some of the factors contributing to their lowered level of violence when compared with the maximum-secure hospitals. There is concern that there has been a loss of skills in dealing with violence in ordinary psychiatric hospitals with the movement of patients either upwards into the secure facilities or into the community and prisons. Most of the medium-secure units which serve large population areas where violence and crime have increased show considerable pressure on beds, thus creating a build up of patients who are potentially difficult to manage, in local psychiatric facilities and the community.

Scotland did not embark on setting up medium-secure units until 1994 (Woodilee Hospital and Levern Hosptial, Glasgow) but did continue to operate locked-ward facilities in addition to the State

Hospital. The main forensic psychiatric base at the Royal Edinburgh Hospital provides training to forensic psychiatrists throughout Scotland along with a unique out-patient forensic psychiatric facility at the Douglas Inch Centre in Glasgow. In recent years the need for development in the east and north-east of Scotland has been recognised with the appointment of a consultant psychiatrist with special forensic interest at the Murray Royal Hospital in Perth and the Royal Cornhill Hospital in Aberdeen, the latter being based on a facility developed over many years by one individual interested in forensic psychiatry.

Facilities for the mentally impaired are provided in two of the Special Hospitals in England (Rampton and Ashworth), and in Carstairs and in Lennox Castle Hospital near Glasgow in Scotland. Lack of predictability is a striking feature of the mentally impaired. As in all Special Hospitals, it is a small number who are responsible for most incidents.

Appendices 1–4

These are given in tabular form on pages 116–121.

Appendix 5. Neuroleptics

Haloperidol

The neuroleptic potency of haloperidol compared with chlorpromazine (CPZ) is 1:50.

Oral dosage. The *British National Formulary* (BNF) recommends 1.5–20 mg daily, gradually increasing to 100 mg (and occasionally 200 mg) in individual doses daily, in severely disturbed patients. Even in the acutely disturbed patient, oral medication should be offered before injection, although it is acknowledged that cooperation can be difficult.

Intramuscular dosage. The BNF recommended dosage for intramuscular injection is 2–10 mg (increasing to 30 mg for emergency control) then 5 mg up to every hour if necessary (intervals of 4–8 hours may be satisfactory).

Intravenous dosage. Haloperidol can be given intravenously and some report little difficulty in obtaining venous access even in disturbed patient. Earlier studies found little advantage in intravenous over oral administration for time of action but it may be that less agitated patients accept oral medicine.

Droperidol

The neuroleptic potency of droperidol compared with CPZ is 2:50.

Oral dosage. A dose of 5–20 mg may be repeated every 4–8 hours if necessary.

Intramuscular dosage. This may be up to 10 mg repeated every 4–6 hours if necessary.

Intravenous dosage. A dose of 5–15 mg may be repeated every 4–6 hours if necessary.

Chlorpromazine

Despite its risks and side-effects, clinicians continue to use chlorpromazine.

Oral dosage. The BNF recommended doses are 25 mg three times daily, adjusted to maintenance of 75–300 mg daily (up to 1 g in psychoses).

Intramuscular dose. A dose of 25–50 mg can be given every 6–8 hours.

Per rectum dose. 100 mg suppository = 20/25 mg intramuscular chlorpromazine.

Sudden death can occur following the intramuscular use of phenothiazines. The cardiotoxic effects and sudden deaths following intramuscular use in struggling patients give cause for caution.

Zuclopenthixol acetate (Acuphase)

This has the same potential for side-effects as other neuroleptics but a different regimen is recommended. The BNF recommended dosage is 50–150 mg (50–100 mg for elderly patients) intramuscularly into gluteal muscle or lateral thigh, repeated if necessary after 2–3 days (one additional dose may be needed 1–2 days after the first injection). The maximum cumulative dose is 400 mg per course (4 injections maximum). If maintenance treatment is necessary, a change to an oral antipsychotic 2–3 days after the last injection is recommended or to a longer-acting antipsychotic depot given with the last injection of zuclopenthixol acetate. This regimen can be tried with violent patients for the short-term management of acute psychosis, mania or exacerbations of chronic psychosis. The main drawback is paradoxically the main benefit – that is, the duration of action – as it can be difficult to stop the action quickly in cases of idiosyncratic response.

References

ANGOLD, A. (1989) Seclusion. *British Journal of Psychiatry*, **154**, 437–444.

BEAN, P., BINGLEY, W., BYNOE, I., et al (1990) *A Place of Safety and Out of Harm's Way*. London: MIND Publications.

BLUGLASS, R. (1992) Editorial. *British Medical Journal*, **305**, 323-324.

BOND, A. & LADER, M. (1979) *Benzodiazepines and Aggression*. pp. 173–182. New York: Raven Press.

CALDWELL, J. & NAISMITH, L. (1989) Violent incidents on special care wards in a special hospital. *Medicine, Science and the Law*, **29**, 116-123.

CAMPBELL, W., SHEPHERD, H. & FALCONER, R. (1982) The use of seclusion. *Nursing Times*, **27**, 1821–1825.

CHAMBERLIN, J. (1985) An ex-patient's response to Soliday. *Journal of Nervous and Mental Disease*, **173**, 288–289.

CONNOLY, J. (1985) *Treatment of the Insane Without Mechanical Restraints*. London: Smith Elder & Co.

CRAFT, M., ISMAIL, I. A., KOISHNAMURTI, D., et al (1987) Lithium in the treatment of aggression in mentally handicapped patients. *British Journal of Psychiatry*, **150**, 685-689.

DEPARTMENT OF HEALTH & WELSH OFFICE (1993) *HMSO Code of Practice. Mental Health Act 1983, Revised 1993*. 18.3–18.30.

DUBIN, W. R. (1988) Rapid tranquilisation: antipsychotics or benzodiazepines? *Journal of Clinical Psychiatry*, (suppl. 49), 5–12.

FOTTRELL, E., BEWLEY, T. & SQUIZZONI, M. (1978) A study of aggressive and violent behaviour. *Medicine, Science and the Law*, **18**, 66-69.

—— (1980) Violence and in-patients in psychiatric hospitals. *British Journal of Psychiatry*, **136**, 216–221.

GENTRY, M. & OSTAPIUK, E. B. (1988) Management of violence in a youth treatment centre. In *Clinical Approaches to Aggression and Violence Issues. Criminological and Legal Psychology*, **12**, 58–68.

GRASSIAN, S. (1983) Psychopathological effects of solitary confinement. *American Journal of Psychiatry*, **140**, 1450–1454.

GREENBERG, A. S. & COLEMAN, M. (1976) Depressed 5-hydroxindole level associated with hyperactive and aggressive behaviour. *Archives of General Psychiatry*, **33**, 331-336.

GUNN, J. & BROWN, J. (1971) Criminality and violence in epileptic patients. *British Journal of Psychiatry*, **118**, 337–343.

GUTHEIL, T. G. (1978) Observations on the theoretical bases for seclusion of the psychiatric inpatient. *American Journal of Psychiatry*, **135**, 325–328.

HODGKINSON, P. (1985) The use of seclusion. *Medicine, Science and the Law*, **25**, 215–222.

HOME OFFICE AND DEPARTMENT OF HEALTH AND SOCIAL SECURITY (1975) *Report of the Committee on Mentally Abnormal Offenders* (Butler report, cmnd 6244). London: HMSO.

HUYSE, F. & STRACK VAN SCHJNDEL, R. (1988) Haloperidol and cardiac arrest. *Lancet*, **ii**, 568–569.

JONES, R. (1988) *Mental Health Act Manual* (2nd edn), pp. 23–24. London: Sweat & Maxwell.

KALOGJERA, I. J., BEDI, A., WATSON, W. N., et al (1989) Impact of therapeutic management on use of seclusion and restraint with disruptive adolescent inpatients. *Hospital and Community Psychiatry*, **40**, 280–285.

KLEGMAN, D. & GOLDBERG, D. A. (1975) Temporal epilepsy and aggression. *Journal of Nervous and Mental Disease*, **160**, 324–341.

LARKIN, E., MURTACH, S. & JONES, S. (1988) A preliminary study of violent incidents in a special hospital (Rampton). *British Journal of Psychiatry*, **153**, 226–231.

LION, J. R., AZCARATE, C. L. & KOEPKE, H. H. (1975) Paradoxical rage reactions during psychotropic medication. *Diseases of the Nervous System*, **36**, 557–558.

Appendix 1. Summary of provisions of the Mental Health Act 1983

Situation	Section	Applicant	Medical recommendation	Duration	Renewal possible
Public place	136	Police constable	–	72 hours	No.
Emergency Community, A&E, Informal patient prior to admission	4	Approved social worker or nearest relative	One medical professional who preferably knows the patient	72 hours	Conversion to section 2 (if applicable) or to section 3
Community, A&E, Informal patient detained under section 4	2	Approved social worker or nearest relative	Two doctors, one of whom knows the patient and one approved by the Secretary of State (section 12)	28 days	No. Conversion to section 3 if applicable
Informal in-patient	5(2)	Registered medical practitioner	–	72 hours	No. Conversion to section 2 or 3
	5(4)	Nurses' holding powers		6 hours	No. Conversion to section 5(2)
Community, A&E, informal in-patient detained under section 2, 4, or 5	3	Approved social worker or nearest relative	Two – one of whom knows the patient and one approved by the Secretary of State	6 months	Yes – after 6 months from date of sections for 6 months; thereafter yearly

A&E, accident and emergency.

Appendix 2. Summary of provisions of the Mental Health (Scotland) Act 1984

Situation	Section	Applicant	Medical recommendation	Duration	Renewal possible	Discharge
Public place	118	Police constable	–	72 hours	No.	Once taken to of place safety
Emergency Community, A&E, informal patient prior to admission	24	Mental health officer, where practicable with consent of nearest relative, inform MWC, nearest relative or person living with the patient as soon as possible	Registered medical practitioner	Admit within 3 days of section	No. Conversion to sections 26 or 18	–
Informal psychiatric in-patient. *Nurses' holding powers*	25	Time and reason for detention recorded in notes. Copied to MWC within 14 days	–	2 hours	No	–
Patient on section 24, informal patient	26	Consent of nearest relative. Managers inform MWC, nearest relative or social worker within 7 days	Medical practitioner approved under section 20	–	No – but can be converted to section 18. Patient can appeal to sheriff for discharge	Yes, by RMO for further 28 days
All above situations	18	Nearest relative who has seen patient within last 14 days. Mental health officer applies to sheriff of patient's residence or if already informal the hospital's sheriff	Two medical recommendations: one approved under section 20; one if practicable by patient's GP. Both to examine within 5 days	Reviews by RMO at one month – 4–6 months, then every year	Yes. Appeals to sheriff by patient	Yes, by RMO, MWC, hospital managers, nearest relative

A&E, accident and emergency; MWC, Mental Welfare Commission; RMO, responsible medical officer.

Appendix 3. Summary of provisions of Part III of the Mental Health Act 1983

Section	Court	Requires	Purpose	Duration	Appeal	Discharge
35	Crown or magistrate	Receiving hospital doctor's oral or written report	Assessment	12 weeks (28 days x 3)	No	–
36	Crown	Two doctors recommending admission	Treatment	12 weeks (28 days x 3)	Can obtain own medical report	–
38	Crown or magistrate	Recommended by 2 registered medical practitioners (1 at hospital receiving patient and 1 approved)	Treatment and assessment of treatability	12 weeks + 28 days x 3 renewals	No	–
37 hospital order	Crown or after conviction at magistrate's court	Recommended by 2 registered medical practitioners (1 at hospital receiving patient and 1 approved)	Treatment	6 months renewable yearly after first 6 months	Patient and nearest relative to MHRT after 6 months, then yearly. Every year must have MHRT	RMO or absent for 28+ days
41 restriction on discharge	Crown	Two registered medical practitioners (1 at hospital receiving patient – 1 must give oral evidence in court but court may invoke even if doctors say no)	Restrict discharge for those who present ongoing risk to public	Unlimited (fixed period becoming rare)	Patient and nearest relative to MHRT after 6 months, thereafter yearly and must have MHRT in 3 years	MHRT or Secretary of State

41 conditional discharge	MHRT or Secretary of State	Discharge plan, usually psychiatric and social	Supervision	Until absolute discharge	Apply to MHRT 12 months after conditional discharge and 2-yearly thereafter	–
47 prison–hospital transfer	Home Secretary	Two registered medical practioners, 1 of whom must be approved under section 12	Treatment	Unlimited or fixed period but becomes notional 37 at expiry of sentence	Patient and nearest relative to MHRT 6 months/1 year after transfer. Must have every 3 years	At expiry of sentence RMO continues detention. MHRT discharge
48	Home Secretary	Two registered medical practitioners, 1 of whom must be approved under section 12	Urgent treatment of remand prisoner	Until trial	MHRT within 6 months, thereafter yearly	Return to prison
49 restriction on discharge	Home Secretary	Two registered medical practitioners	Restriction on discharge	Until date of release from prison	MHRT within 6 months	–

RMO, responsible medical officer; MHRT, mental health review tribunal.

Appendix 4. Summary of provisions of Part VI of the Mental Health (Scotland) Act 1984

Legal status	Type of order	Requirement	Duration/outcome	Renewal	Appeal	Discharge
Before trial at sheriff or High Court (district court must refer to higher court)	Transfer order (section 70)	Two doctors, 1 of whom is approved under section 20	Until trial or sentence	–	Within 1 month of transfer. Appeal to sheriff	If appeal succeeds remit to prison; RMO may discharge back to prison
Before trial at sheriff or High Court (district court must refer to higher court)	Insane on bar of trial: Criminal Procedures Scotland Act 1975	Two doctors, 1 of whom is approved under section 20	State Hospital Carstairs or "another"	Indefinite annual reports	"Defence" psychiatrist appeal to sheriff of origin or Secretary of State	By sheriff or Secretary of State, *not* managers or RMO
Insane at time of offence	Insane at time of offence	Jury finds insane at time of offence (no retrial possible)	State Hospital Carstairs or "another"	Indefinite annual reports	Appeal to sheriff or Secretary of State	By sheriff or Secretary of State, *not* managers or RMO
Convicted at sheriff or High Court	Interim hospital order	Two doctors, 1 of whom is approved under section 20	Three months in State Hospital or another hospital if there is a special reason	Every 28 days until 6 months in total	Once in 6-month period	–

Convicted at sheriff or High Court	Remand on bail	Court plus acceptance by hospital	Three weeks	Three weeks	None	–
Convicted at sheriff or High Court	Hospital order (section 60)	Two doctors, 1 of whom is approved under section 20	Admit within 28 days	After 4–6 months; thereafter annually	To sheriff	By RMO or MWC, *not* nearest relative
Risk to public. Serious offence history	Restriction order (section 62)	Two doctors, 1 of whom is approved under section 20, one to give oral evidence	Time limited (rare) or indefinite	Annual report by RMO	To sheriff after first 6 months and annually	By sheriff or Secretary of State; absolute or conditional
Sentenced prisoner. Civil prisoner (debtor). People detained under Immigration Act 1971	Transfer direction (section 72) (same effect as hospital order and/or restriction direction)	Two doctors, 1 of whom is approved under section 20	Lasts as long as sentence	Report by RMO within 28 days of expiry of sentence. Converts to a hospital order	Within one month to sheriff	Remitted to original prison. If no report is made patient is automatically discharged at expiry of date of sentence

RMO, responsible medical officer; MWC, Mental Welfare Commission.

Times (1988) Lord Keith in the case of Black v Forsey *et al*, 1987. SLT 681. *Times*, 21 May.

Mullen, P. E. (1988) Violence and mental disorder. *British Journal of Hospital Medicine*, **40**, 460–463.

Pilowsky, L. S., Ring, H., Shine, P. J., *et al* (1992) Rapid tranquillisation. *British Journal of Psychiatry*, **160**, 831–835.

Plutchik, R., Karasu, T. B., Conte, H. R., *et al* (1978) Toward a rationale for the seclusion process. *Journal of Nervous and Mental Disease*, **166**, 571.

Russell, D., Hodgkinson, P. & Hillis, T. (1986) Time out: are disturbed patients secluded for purely clinical reasons? *Nursing Times*, 26 February, 47–49.

Sheard, M. H. (1984) Clinical pharmacology of aggressive behaviour. *Clinical Neuropharmacology*, **7**, 173-183.

Soliday, S. M. (1985) A comparison of patient and staff attitudes towards seclusion. *Journal of Nervous and Mental Disease*, **173**, 273–286.

Sorgi, P. J., Ratey, J. J. & Polakoff, S. (1986) Beta-adrenergic blockers for the control of aggressive behaviours in patients with chronic schizophrenia. *American Journal of Psychiatry*, **143**, 775–776.

Tardiff, K. & Sweillam, A. (1982) Assaultive behaviour among chronic in-patients. *American Journal of Psychiatry*, **139**, 212–215.

Taylor, P. J. (1985) Motives for offending among violent and psychotic men. *British Journal of Psychiatry*, **147**, 491-498.

—— & Gunn, J. (1984) Violence and psychosis. *British Medical Journal*, **288**, 1945–1949.

Tupin, J. P. (1978) Lithium for aggressiveness (letter). *American Journal of Psychiatry*, **135**, 1118.

—— (1983) The violent patient: a strategy for management and diagnosis. *Hospital and Community Psychiatry*, **34**, 61.

Turks, E. R. & Dermen, S. W. (1977) Carbamazepine in the dyscontrol syndrome associated with limbic system dysfunction. *Journal of Nervous and Mental Disease*, **164**, 56–63.

Wadeson, H. & Carpenter, W. T. (1976) Impact of the seclusion room experience. *Journal of Nervous and Mental Disease*, **163**, 318–328.

6   Role of the organisation

CAMERON STARK and BRIAN KIDD

The significance of violence to an organisation

Violence towards staff is an important issue for any organisation. For health care organisations, where a safe environment is essential for the effective delivery of care, threats and assaults take on an even greater importance. Problems arise when any degree of violence is accepted as normal, whether directed towards staff or clients. Violence can result in a spiral, with staff injury and distress resulting in time off work; staff taking increased sick leave; overtime costs for staff cover increasing; avoidance of some clients with consequent reduction of effectiveness; and a loss of confidence in the organisation (Scott & Whitehead, 1981).

Many factors conspire to reduce the profile of violence. Assaults resulting in serious injury are rare. If the organisation views them as unusual events then there seems little point in expending time, effort and money in trying to prevent them. In addition, it is easy for organisations to regard serious assaults as isolated incidents. When such events do occur, they provide a focus for pre-existing staff concerns, and may legitimise discussion of violence, allowing staff to reveal their worries. Managers may be unprepared for the degree of feeling displayed in the aftermath of serious or potentially serious incidents, and the concerns may prompt a brief, sticking-plaster response, with measures aimed solely at the cause of the event, and the issue then falling into an uneasy quiet until the next incident occurs. In this way, many health care units react to violence rather than planning how to address and prevent it in advance.

Another factor interfering with a systematic approach to the problem is an awareness that if violence is acknowledged as a problem, then it becomes necessary to accept responsibility for its prevention. Some staff and managers accept the concept of the 'deserving victim', which absolves units of the need to investigate incidents thoroughly, and removes accountability. Managers are often accused of taking this stance, but the position also has attractions to staff. If a person can be assaulted and injured or killed through no fault of their own, then any staff member is vulnerable. This is an uncomfortable realisation and staff, as well as managers, may prefer to believe that the victim is different from themselves by virtue of some act of commission or omission which resulted in the assault. Managers should be aware that staff may have complicated feelings about violence, related to their own vulnerabilities, and which may affect the management of change.

Staff safety should not be seen as a separate issue from security as a whole. The cost of theft in the National Health Service (NHS) is extraordinary, and its reduction has been seen as a priority by the NHS Executive (Yarrow 1993*a,b*). Many of the approaches designed to increase staff safety are equally applicable to the reduction of pilfering. Recent highly publicised cases of neonatal kidnapping, which could happen as easily in psychiatric units with mother-and-baby facilities as in general or maternity hospitals, also lend extra weight to other simple recommendations, including the use of name badges (Friend, 1991; *Health Service Journal*, 1994).

Legal requirements

> "All employers have a legal duty under Section 2(1) of the Health and Safety at Work Act 1974 to ensure, so far as is reasonably practicable, the health, safety and welfare of their employees. This duty can extend to protecting employees from assaults." (Health and Safety Executive, 1989)

This responsibility has been reinforced by the Management of Health and Safety at Work Regulations 1992, which came into force in January 1993. These regulations, based on a European Community directive, are intended to make more explicit the requirements of the 1974 Act. They require employers:

(a) to assess the risks to the health and safety of their employees, and of anyone else who may be affected by their work activity
(b) to record any significant findings, if the organisation has more than five employees
(c) to arrange to put steps following on from this assessment into practice; this has to cover planning, organisation, control, monitoring and review
(d) to allocate competent people, either from within their organisation, or outside it, to help them formulate and implement the necessary measures
(e) to establish emergency procedures

(f) to ensure that employees have "adequate health and safety training, and are capable enough at their job to avoid risks" (Health and Safety Commission, 1992).

The Health and Safety Executive makes it clear that the employer has an important role to play in ensuring that the employee is working in as safe a working environment as is possible. There seems little doubt that these regulations apply to violence as well as to other, more recognised, health and safety at work issues (Stark & Paterson, 1994).

As was recognised in the Skelmersdale report (Department of Health and Social Security, 1988), in some work situations employees will be at high risk of exposure to violence or aggression by virtue of the fact that they are dealing with the general public. There may also be specific situations or work settings where clients are recognised as being more dangerous or the staff more at risk. For example, in health care the areas of accident and emergency medicine, community health, and psychiatry have been particularly associated with violence. There are no available statistics which support the notion that any area of health care is entirely without risk. There appears to be a spectrum of risk to staff working with the public, and employers must examine the question of violence towards all its employees appropriately, tapering their approach to each work setting, each occupational group and even each individual.

In keeping with the regulations, organisations should tackle the following areas:

(a) identification of the extent of the problem
(b) establishing and maintaining an efficient monitoring and reporting system; this must include a clear definition of violence, allowing the classification of all events
(c) looking at the working environment with a view to prevention or at least reduction of violent incidents
(d) establishing and maintaining a system of post-incident support and counselling
(e) initiating appropriate training in aggression management for all staff, adapted to the needs of individual groups of workers
(f) maintaining an organisational commitment to the topic, with an emphasis on prevention.

These areas overlap. For example, training may incorporate issues about reporting of incidents, and efficient monitoring allows a clear identification of the extent of the problem. It is valuable to examine each area individually, but it is important that there is an individual who is responsible for coordinating matters related to violence at work. This named individual should have the monitoring of violence and the organisation of training programmes as identified objectives, which should be regularly assessed. A manager may delegate many of the tasks, but it should be clear with whom responsibility for the programme rests.

Identification of the extent of the problem

How does an employer determine the extent of the problem? The Health and Safety Executive (1989) recommends that the easiest way to find out if there is a problem in the workplace is to "ask your staff". While there are problems with definitions and reporting biases, as discussed further below, this has the advantage of simplicity. It can be done by formal surveys, small-group discussion, or by listening to comments while 'walking the job'. It may also help to empower staff to consider the topic by letting them know that it is taken seriously, and that management are interested in their views, and acknowledge their skills, expertise and experience.

The consequence of seeking information will be a raising of expectations, and if the organisation embarks on this process it should be prepared to make efforts to feed results back to staff, and to demonstrate evidence of an appropriate response to the findings. The result of canvassing views and experiences without subsequent action will be to make staff cynical and disillusioned. In these circumstances encouraging participation a second time will be that much more difficult.

Information

Routine information sources are an important part of the process of assessing the prevalence of violence. Incident report forms, accident reports and sick leave may all give clues to prevalence, but are likely to paint an incomplete picture. Up to 80% of assaults may be unreported (Lion *et al*, 1981; Kidd & Stark, 1992), while very few instances of verbal abuse will find their way into formal records. Accident report forms are often completed for only the most serious incidents, or for those thought to have resulted in injury. Incident report forms, used in many hospitals and community units, may be a better guide, as breakages, physical assaults or episodes in which clients were physically restrained may be included. Other health care units ask only that nursing staff record the names of clients involved in 'special incidents', often with no indication of the nature of the episode.

It will be necessary to combine information from different sources to compile a profile of violence in an organisation. In general, existing records will give more insight into serious incidents than into violence as a whole. If this inverse pyramid with disproportionate reporting of serious incidents is recognised, then the use of overlapping data sources can be used to make some estimate of prevalence. An ad hoc survey of nursing notes, carried out by an audit officer or administrative assistant, will offer information on episodes which do not reach the staff's threshold for completion of a formal incident report.

If an organisation wishes to have a detailed view of less serious incidents, a prospective study will be necessary. This can be done by encouraging detailed data collection over a short period – a few weeks or months – in a ward or unit. The site (or sites) can be chosen either because of local concern, or to reflect a cross-section of the organisation's activities. The process of data collection will be affected by the factors influencing reporting discussed below, and by the concentration on a particular area. This has to be carefully managed to avoid staff feeling that their ward or unit has been selected because of concerns about their performance.

The information collected from such an exercise can be helpful in detailed planning, but the effort expended may be better invested in improving the quality of routine information collecting.

Assessing risk

The range of experience needed to assess and interpret all risks is unlikely to be found in a single person, and a group process is usually required. To encourage ownership of both problems and solutions, it is helpful to involve a range of staff from the outset. The decision to examine security will often follow from an incident which has caused concern in the organisation. In such a situation, it is particularly important that the group carries out an assessment of the risks, as well as the potential solutions, or one or two high-profile incidents may overshadow less obvious, but no less important threats.

The group should include a manager of sufficient seniority to demonstrate the organisation's commitment to prevention and management of violence. This manager will often chair the group. Clinical service managers or their equivalent can also usefully be included, and it is essential to have a contribution from staff working directly in contact with clients. In large organisations, occupational health staff are also likely to be involved. The aim of the process has to be to produce an assessment and solution which is seen as relevant and helpful by the staff who will have to implement it, and the make-up of the group can do much to aid this.

It is necessary for the group to be clear on organisational aims. For example, if the unit or organisation aims to deliver care only in one site within office hours, then this focuses attention much more than with a unit which intends to provide community care using workers detached from their base. Once organisational aims are explicitly stated, it will be apparent what areas need to be reviewed. A clear statement should also be made of who is to be safeguarded – clients, staff and public, for example. The personnel who will deliver care, and the environment in which it will be delivered, should then be defined (see case example 6.1). Ishimoto (1984) suggests that threats in each environment should be listed and known vulnerabilities (from accident report forms, etc.) discussed.

Case example 6.1

After a violent incident, a psychiatric social work service, operating within a mental health campus in the grounds of an old hospital wanted to examine its procedures for the management of violence. A client had become aggressive while waiting for a delayed appointment. The person had left the waiting-room, entered a clerical office and shouted at the secretary. The receptionist sounded an alarm buzzer (fitted two years before, after another episode). A social worker had come from another office to find out the cause of the noise. By the time anyone called the police the episode had grown to such an extent that a window was broken and secretary, receptionist and social worker were all greatly distressed. A small group, consisting of the assistant manager, two social workers and a receptionist, was formed. They agreed that the aim of the organisation was to deliver a service: during office hours within their unit; to wards and clinics on the hospital site, again within office hours; and to clients in the community, often outside normal hours. Looking first at the office, the initial area of concern, they agreed that the staff involved included social workers, secretarial and reception staff and potentially police. Their aim was to protect clients, staff and any other members of the public (such as relatives) who might be present. Looking at other reported episodes, and drawing on their experience and that of others in their department, they listed the vulnerabilities, including clients in the waiting-room, corridors and offices. Other threats included the appointment system, which often resulted in clients waiting for up to an hour. The receptionist felt she had to defend the social work staff, and did not usually explain the cause for the delay. The lack of staff training in how to respond to an alert was another obvious threat. The receptionist and secretary recounted a similar episode from a few months before. This had been less serious, and no formal record of it had been made, nor action taken. The recommendations from the working group were that the appointment procedure be altered, and waiting times audited. The receptionist was to keep clients notified of the waiting time, and to explain the cause for the delay wherever possible. Social workers would help by keeping the receptionist informed of likely delays. The group identified the secretarial office as being a staff area, for which patient access was not necessary. Recommendations were made for staff to record incidents and to discuss them at the monthly department meetings. Three months later, the appointment system was running more smoothly. An electronic number lock, costing less than £100, had been fitted to the secretarial office. Mock alerts had been held twice since the group reported. These had brought further problems to the fore, and the department was seeking funds to send the receptionist and some of the social workers on a course to learn calming and de-escalation techniques.

Definitions and monitoring

The organisation has to have a clear definition of violence if its prevalence is to be monitored. Breakwell has discussed possible definitions in Chapter 1. The use of different criteria to define a violent incident in different organisations causes problems for researchers, and makes cross-organisation comparisons difficult. This problem is of secondary importance to those tackling violence in a specific setting: their priority must be clear, acceptable definitions which make sense to those who will apply them. Many workplaces will want to provide definitions for other problems, such as bullying or sexual harassment at work. These other types of violence are outside the scope of this volume.

Whether definitions are developed or used from elsewhere, the system used should include a classification of the type of incident (physical assault, verbal abuse, etc.) and a measure of severity. The British Medical Association (1993) defines violence as:

> "The application of force, severe threat or serious abuse, by members of the public towards people arising out of the course of their work whether or not they are on duty . . . . [this includes] Severe verbal abuse or threat where this is judged likely to turn into actual violence: serious or persistent harassment (including racial or sexual harassment); threat with a weapon; major or minor injuries; fatalities."

This definition includes verbal abuse and persistent harassment, both of which may be accepted by employees as part of the job. The Health and Safety Executive (1989) taxonomy includes a measurement of severity (Table 6.1).

TABLE 6.1

The Health and Safety Executive's classification of violent incidents

Type of incident	Result
Involving physical contact	Fatal injury Major injury Injury or emotional shock requiring first aid, out-patient treatment, counselling, absence from work (*record number of days*)
Involving serious or persistent threats or verbal abuse	Emotional shock requiring counselling or absence from work (*record number of days*); feeling of being at risk or under great stress

Failure to report

Violent incidents in hospitals often go unreported. Lion *et al* (1981) found only 17% of incidents were reported, similar to the 20% reporting indicated in the Health and Safety Executive (1989) report. Other studies have reported similar findings.

Reasons for staff failing to report incidents include:

(a) lack of available guidelines or operational policy or lack of knowledge of these guidelines/policies (Whitfield & Shelley, 1991; Kidd & Stark, 1992)

(b) no (or inadequate) form for recording incidents

(c) time and effort required to fill in report

(d) staff perceive violence as 'part of the job'

(e) concern that a violent incident will be perceived as 'performance failure'

(f) fear of litigation.

Case example 6.2

A community trust, which included mental health services, was concerned about incomplete reporting of violent incidents. The management team consulted clinical staff and designed new guidelines for the management of violent incidents, together with a new reporting form. All wards were supplied with a copy of the guidelines, together with one copy of the reporting form. Each ward was expected to make further copies of the form for their own use. No guidance on completion of the forms was given, and ward staff often did not know the reason for the exercise. In many wards few if any further copies were made. When copies were used, the original form was often used to report incidents happening at night or at weekends, when it was not possible to copy further forms. After an initial increase in reporting, the level of incidents recorded fell below the numbers which had caused the initial concern about under-reporting. The changes had been well intentioned, but good preparatory work was let down by lack of attention to detail.

Case example 6.3

An education department introduced a rigorous new reporting and evaluation procedure for violence at work: if an incident occurred in a residential institution, the establishment was visited by a three-person inspection team. The investigation took up to three working days, and all staff and clients were interviewed. The emphasis was on discovering 'what had gone wrong'. The episode was recorded in the staff member's personnel file. A striking drop in reports was taken as evidence of the success of prevention policies. Anecdotal reports suggested that episodes still occurred, but were not reported. The organisation lost the opportunity to benefit from open discussion of episodes, by making the procedure too top heavy.

To enhance reporting, there must be clear guidelines about what incidents should be reported, and this should be based on the concerns of staff. A simple form, easy to use, should be readily available to all staff. Examples of standard forms are available from the Health and Safety Executive. Staff should be made aware of these provisions and their use should be regularly reviewed. This exercise could also be incorporated into the audit activities of a unit, with comparisons of reports being compared with the documented violence in case files, nursing notes and so on, as discussed above. In this way a clear record of the employees' exposure to violence can be gathered and used to gauge the effectiveness of training, environmental changes or other measures to reduce risk to staff.

Establishing a fully functioning reporting system has many benefits. It allows continuous monitoring of the extent of the problem, and identifies potential weak spots in the working systems. It also supplies information to professionals working with the same clients, alerting them to any potential dangers.

The organisation must not assume that a monitoring system will be used simply because it exists. Establishing such a system can be seen as the first step in increasing awareness of violent incidents, but will not be successful if not supported in other ways. For example, staff must have confidence in the system, being sure that reporting an incident will not automatically result in the attachment of blame. Instead, a commitment to the reporting system must be fostered so that staff members can understand the likely benefits, to themselves and others, of collecting this information. This requires a continuing programme of feedback, education and training.

Environmental issues

Location of incidents

It is important to consider the influence of the environment, both in reducing the likelihood of violence occurring, and in making it easier to manage when it happens. In general practice, the surgery is the most common location for violence to occur. In one study, 41% of incidents in general practice were associated with long waiting times (Hobbs, 1991). The British Medical Association General Medical Services Committee (1993) surveyed general practitioners in London and found that 87% of threats and 68.4% of assaults took place in the surgery.

Attention to details in the waiting-room may reduce the tendency to violence. In psychiatry, where patients are often under considerable psychological stress and may be psychotic, the patient may have to wait in a drab waiting-room and be interviewed in an isolated, cramped office, which may increase the likelihood both of violence and of an incident resulting in injury. Although assaults in the community are of great concern, many of the most publicised assaults on staff have occurred in health care premises. The murder of social worker Isabel Schwarz, which led to the Spokes report and a far-reaching review of social workers' safety, took place inside a psychiatric hospital, as did the murder of Georginal Robinson, an occupational therapist (Blom-Cooper *et al*, 1995).

In the area of social work and community nursing, much of the work is in the community, and in this setting the problem of staff isolation may have its own effect on the possible severity of violent incidents. This may be further worsened by the fact that (in social work) at the fieldwork level women outnumber men and may therefore be more vulnerable (Norris, 1990).

Altering the environment

The Health and Safety Executive (1989) saw the working environment as one of the key areas which could be altered to help prevent violence. Issues such as design of waiting-rooms, layout of seating, room lighting, colour of walls and activities to alleviate boredom may have an influence on potential aggressors. They made some specific suggestions. Reception areas should be well signposted and freely accessible. Lighting should be diffuse and glare free and also bright enough to light all areas, leaving no dark corners. Client areas should be spacious enough to allow people not to feel cramped or hemmed in. Sources of noise should be minimised (e.g. banging doors or squeaking trolleys) and sound-absorbing surfaces should be used where possible. Wall coverings should be in subdued colours and adroit use of plants and pictures can produce a peaceful, homely environment. A good choice of magazines and reading material can alleviate boredom, as can televisions and provision of toys, taking into account the potential for noise. Vending machines and telephone access enable clients to communicate with others, and to obtain refreshments without leaving the waiting area and risking missing their appointment. Seating should be durable but comfortable and in good repair. Fittings should always be chosen to minimise the opportunity to use them as a weapon.

Security

Controlling access to particular sites and ensuring adequate monitoring of sites are both important issues to consider (Hall, 1993). It is often necessary to review the physical layout of a department. Once the organisational aims are clarified, it is possible to decide which areas are client areas and which are for staff only, and at what times of the day (a ward may operate free visiting during the day, but not be open to access from outside at night, when there are fewer staff and clients are more vulnerable).

The flow of clients within a department can also be considered. For example, if there are several entrances and exits to a department, it will be much more difficult to keep track of where clients are located than if there is only one way in or out which is in view of a receptionist (Morse & Morse, 1984). Redirecting flow by closing an entrance can often be effective. This may lead on to consideration of the design of client areas, particularly reception and waiting areas. Accident and emergency departments now avoid having 'blind spots', and this can be emulated in all health care reception areas. Often, moving a reception desk or installing a mirror will allow all of an area to become visible.

Technological aides can also be considered. Site access can be limited by electronic locks, opened by typing in numbers on a key pad, or by 'swipe' cards, run through a slot in the lock. These are useful, but may be impractical where rapid access by staff in an emergency is essential. Similarly, electronic surveillance with closed-circuit television (CCTV) may be a useful aide. CCTV can allow one individual to monitor many areas at once, and timed video recordings allow movements at entrances and exits to be timed. The introduction of smaller cameras using new technology which does not involve cathode-ray tubes has made systems less obtrusive and often cheaper. Simultaneous recordings can be made from many cameras on to one video tape, but later viewed individually if required (Cole & McKee, 1993). These systems have a place in an overall security system, but seldom allow constant monitoring of all areas.

Alarm systems are often discussed after particularly serious incidents. Again, they can be a useful part of an integrated response, but cannot be a solution in themselves. There are various forms of alarm systems, with the most versatile using alarms carried on the person to communicate with local remote units which relay the alarm back to a central point. Many security companies now offer products and services to the health care sector, and are happy to offer advice and tender for systems.

Relationships with the local police force are important. Problems in the day-to-day relationship between police force and health care workers usually arise from misunderstandings and prejudices. Police officers may be reluctant to attend incidents in hospitals because of a belief that violence invariably results as a consequence of mental illness, and that health care staff should be able to handle them in isolation. This can also produce a reluctance to prosecute clients of a mental health service, as officers may feel that, by virtue of their contact with a psychiatric service, the person is absolved of any responsibility for their actions.

On the other side of this potential divide, health care staff often believe that the police force will be insensitive in their approach, and prone to blame staff or treat clients poorly. The myths on each side grow in isolation, and affect other parts of mental health services, such as police referrals for emergency assessment. Rosenheck (1985) demonstrated that joint discussions and mutual education can do much to overcome these barriers.

Organisations may conclude that, even with improved relations with the police, changes to the environment and improved staff training, it will still not be possible to deal with all security matters. Some decide to employ security guards. These can be employed directly by the organisation, or the service contracted out to a specialist security organisation. The decision to proceed with such a step is an important one, and the merits of employing guards can be discussed with the local police force and the various companies which offer commercial security services. Contracting out the service can save money, but may produce problems with lack of control over staff, and with reduced flexibility in staff duties.

Establishing/maintaining a system of post-incident support and counselling

The Health Services Advisory Committee (1987) highlighted the possible effects of violence towards professionals who "are accustomed to being helpers not being helped" and suggested that "some individuals may need support and counselling, especially on return to work". Organisations should ensure that post-incident support is available to all staff who need it.

While it is essential that all employers supply post-incident support for staff, this should not include 'victim blaming' and should incorporate a sympathetic approach to staff exposed to violence. This would help to avoid such incidents as the sacking of a midwife for allegedly "failing to stay calm" when threatened by a hospital visitor (*Health Service Journal*, 1992). The details of the provision of post-incident support are discussed in Chapter 7.

Initiating appropriate training

Infantino & Musingo (1985) demonstrated that staff trained in the management of verbal and physical aggression were less likely to be injured by violence at work. Carmel & Hunter (1990) replicated this work, and produced similar findings. They compared wards where a high proportion of staff had been trained with wards where few staff had been trained. The two groups of wards did not differ on other characteristics. Both groups of wards experienced the same number of violent incidents, but staff in the wards where training was common were less likely to sustain an injury. The information required to assess the cost-effectiveness of training is currently unavailable. The available evidence, however, suggests that training decreases injuries and probably reduces time off work. It can also be expected to improve staff morale and to emphasise an organisation's commitment to quality.

There is little evidence to allow comparison of different training strategies. Leadbetter and Paterson, however, identify the components which can be included in a comprehensive training programme (Chapter 4). Their list is formidable, but this does not mean that all staff must be trained in all of the skills. Rather, they should have the ability to cope with the degree of violence to which they are likely to be exposed. It is evident that some areas of work are more dangerous than others. Also, different professions are likely to be confronted with violence in different ways and with differing effects. It is therefore essential that training is tapered to the employees' needs in a particular work setting (Stark & Kidd, 1994).

(a) A secretary who works in an office and has no direct contact with a client other than by telephone may not be exposed to physical violence but is likely to be exposed to verbal violence. Her training would be expected to take this into account and would entail basic instruction in office security, some advice on personal safety, and advice and practice in dealing with aggressive telephone callers.

(b) A librarian working alone in a satellite library in an inner city area is very likely to be exposed to verbal and physical threats as well as people causing damage to property. Training in this instance would entail basic security and personal safety, as above. The librarian would also require training in de-escalation techniques and, given that he/she were working in isolation, training in breakaway techniques.

(c) A nurse working in an intensive-care unit within a psychiatric hospital works with clients who may be placed in the ward because of violent behaviour. Staff in the unit would be expected to provide care and to protect clients from both themselves and others. Training in this instance would include the hospital security, personal safety, de-escalation and break-away training mentioned above. The nurse would also require training in defusing, and control and restraint techniques.

Maintaining an organisational commitment

It is common for an emergency or serious assault to focus attention on the issue, for changes to be made in response, and the matter then to fall from organisational agendas. One of the key roles of the organisation is in maintaining commitment to the prevention and management of violence.

It is possible to make use of reporting systems to maintain the momentum towards change, and to reinforce the importance of reporting accuracy. If report forms are collated and the anonymised information circulated throughout the unit (e.g. number and type of incidents over a set period), then staff have evidence of some of the uses to which the information is put, and of the importance their managers attach to the issue.

Similarly, a serious assault or potentially serious breakdown in procedures can be used to reinforce commitment rather than be taken as an indication that the efforts made have failed. Establishing

Summary points

- Organisations often review safety procedures after a violent incident. This can be valuable, but should be part of a measured and consistent approach to the problem.
- Health and safety regulations make it clear that employers must assess risks to their staff, and take steps to minimise the risk from the hazards they identify. Employers who do not make a thorough assessment of risks of assault, and act on those findings, may be challenged in court.
- The organisational response to occupational violence should include: review of the extent and nature of the problem; establishment of an effective monitoring system; identification of training and security needs; establishment of a post-incident support and review system; continuing organisational commitment.
- Training in the prevention and management of violent incidents can be targeted on those most at need of training, and extended to other staff as resources permit. This will require a training needs assessment for all staff groups.
- Training is only one component of the necessary response, which should include the installation and maintenance of physical security measures identified by the overall needs assessment.
- Organisational policies should demonstrate continued commitment to the prevention and management of violence.

a system for the review of this type of critical incident, with involvement of clinical staff, trainers and managers, should allow adverse events to act as an opportunity to examine policies and to fine-tune them without having to discard what has gone before.

The type of debriefing techniques developed for use after major emergencies will often prove useful. In such debriefing sessions, normal divisions of rank are put aside, and the independent chairperson makes it clear that it is not an opportunity to offer personal criticisms or settle old scores. The chairperson prepares an agenda in advance and takes the group through a detailed examination of the incident, including its repercussions on policy and planning. The aim of such a meeting must be to learn without causing further distress to those involved. This type of response, if carried out effectively, should encourage staff participation in any future debriefings and have the effect of emphasising the importance the organisation places on the welfare of the staff.

Conclusions

Preventing and managing violence is important to an organisation, and should be regarded as an indication of quality. Assessing the problem requires involvement of all staff. Maintaining interest in the problem needs considerable organisational commitment and managerial attention. The difficulties in addressing violence should not be underestimated, but they are balanced by the potential benefits.

References

BLOM-COOPER, L., HALLY, H. & MURPHY, E. (1995) *The Falling Shadow: One Patient's Mental Health Care 1978–93.* London: Duckworth.

BRITISH MEDICAL ASSOCIATION GENERAL MEDICAL SERVICES COMMITTEE (1993) *Confidential Survey of London GPs: Final Report.* London: Electoral Reform Ballot Services.

CARMEL, H. & HUNTER, M. (1990) Compliance with training in managing assaultive behaviour and injuries from in-patient violence. *Hospital and Community Psychiatry,* **41**, 558–560.

COLE, T. & McKEE, M. (1993) Keeping a watchful eye with closed-circuit TV. In *British Hospital Management.* pp 221–223. London, Sterling.

DEPARTMENT OF HEALTH AND SOCIAL SECURITY (1988) *Report of the DHSS Advisory Committee on Violence to Saff. Chairperson: Lord Skelmersdale.* London: HMSO.

FRIEND, B. (1991) Security: a lesson learnt. *Nursing Times,* **87**, 35.

HALL, D. (1993) Effective security for hospitals. In *British Hospital Management.* pp 207–210. London: Sterling.

HEALTH AND SAFETY COMMISSION (1992) Management of health and safety at work: approved code of practice. *Management of Health and Safety at Work Regulations 1992.* London: HMSO.

HEALTH AND SAFETY EXECUTIVE (1989) *Violence to Staff* (IND(G) 1\89 M100). London: HMSO.

HEALTH AND SAFETY ADVISORY COMMITTEE (1987) *Violence to Staff in the Health Services.* DHSS Advisory Committee on Violence to Staff Report. London: DHSS.

HEALTH SERVICE JOURNAL (1992) Staff back sacked and abused midwife. *Health Service Journal,* 2 April, 7.

HEALTH SERVICE JOURNAL (1994) Better safe than sorry. *Health Service Journal,* 21 July, 15.

HOBBS, F. D. R. (1991) Violence in general practice: a survey of general practitioners' views. *British Medical Journal,* **302**, 329–332.

INFANTINO, J. A. JR. & MUSINGO, S. Y. (1985) Assaults and injuries among staff with and without training in aggression control techniques. *Hospital and Community Psychiatry*, **36**, 1312– 1314.

ISHIMOTO, W. (1984) Security management for health care administrators. In *Violence in the Medical Care Setting* (ed. J. T. Turner). Rockville: Aspen.

KIDD, B. & STARK, C. (1992) Violence and junior doctors working in psychiatry. *Psychiatric Bulletin*, **16**, 144–145.

LION, J. R., SNYDER W. & MERRILL, G. L. (1981) Under-reporting of assaults on staff in a state hospital. *Hospital and Community Psychiatry*, **32**, 497–498.

MORSE, G. P. & MORSE, R. F. (1984) Protection overlooked in hospital design. *Hospitals*, **58**, 78.

NORRIS, D. (1990) *Violence Against Social Workers: the Implications for Practice.* London: Jessica Kingsley.

ROSENHECK, R. (1985) From conflict to collaboration: psychiatry and the hospital police. *Psychiatry*, **48**, 254–263.

SCOTT, J. R. & WHITEHEAD, J. J. (1981) An administrative approach to the problem of violence. *Journal of Mental Health Administration*, **8**, 36–40.

STARK, C. & KIDD, B. (1995) Assessment of training needs in the prevention and management of violence. *Advanced Hospital Management* (in press).

—— & PATERSON, B. (1994) Violence at work. *British Medical Journal*, **308**, 62–63.

WHITFIELD, W. & SHELLEY, P. (1991) Violence and the CPN: a survey. *Community Psychiatric Nursing Journal*, 13–17.

YARROW, S. (1993*a*) The Crook report. *Health Service Journal*, 20 May, 14.

—— (1993*b*) Climate of fear. Crime in the NHS Special Report. *Health Service Journal* (suppl. 103), 1–2.

7 Post-incident care and support for assaulted staff

ERICA ROBB

Most of us picture our world as inherently safe. For professionals working with difficult or violent clients, this belief is necessary to allow us to go to work each day able to assume that we will not be constantly under threat of injury or harm. Janoff-Bulman & Frieze (1983) postulated that we require three basic assumptions to allow us to manage our lives comfortably:

(a) a belief in our own personal invulnerability
(b) seeing the world we inhabit as fair and predictable
(c) having positive confidence in our ability to cope with challenges.

Belief in the protection from assault that our own worth provides and belief in our skill in using caution to prevent misfortune are also important.

Assault by a client or a member of a client's family throws such assumptions and beliefs about our safety into disarray and forces us to re-examine and reconstruct the framework or schemata by which we judge our world. It takes time to manage the new and sudden concepts that we are no longer inviolate and that our world has become dangerous, threatening and unpredictable. There is also anger and resentment that anyone, particularly someone for whom we feel professionally responsible, could treat us with malevolence and aggression, and the inevitable question of why we were chosen to be the victim in this instance – were we culpable in some way?

The attribution of blame for the assault is an important factor in the management of staff who are assaulted. For staff caring for others there is another basic personal belief which is challenged when an assault occurs, and that is the belief that they are in control of the situation and can manage their clients effectively. Disruption of this assumption can cause doubt in their confidence as a capable professional, guilt and self-blame. Lanza (1985) reviewed the literature on staff assault and found a tendency to place blame on the nurse for a patient's assault on that nurse. Clearly, the way in which managers deal with their staff who are the victims of an assault can assist such staff to apportion blame appropriately and understand that there are certain situations which cannot always be planned for or prevented.

Conn & Lion (1983) found in a study of the psychological consequences of physical assault on psychiatric staff that "almost unanimously the victims of assault agreed that the emotional impact of being attacked far exceeded the impact of physical injury".

Ryan & Poster (1989) studied 61 staff who had been assaulted by their patients, where assault was defined as physical contact with intent to harm or physical contact by a patient opposing restraint procedures. They found that 67% had significant responses to the incident within one week but that most staff felt that they had dealt with their reaction to the assault by the sixth week. Some of the staff, however, had a delayed reaction 6–12 months afterwards. The strongest responses were in the emotional and physiological categories, including anger, anxiety and increased muscle tension. These staff victims also reported compassion for their assailant and a feeling that they could have prevented the attack.

An assault is thus a stressful and violent disruption of our daily lives which can throw us off balance in a way which means that our whole approach to life is changed – an experience which forms the basis for the development of post-traumatic stress disorder. The implication of this is that if people are assaulted, it is important that they are able to come to terms with what has happened in a way that helps them to adapt positively and which will inoculate them against future stress by providing them with understanding and successful coping strategies. Depending on how the reconstruction of our basic system of beliefs about ourselves in relation to our world occurs, our future assumptions and the moods and feelings which arise from such beliefs can lead to positive adaptation for more successful coping strategies or negative avoidance and maladaptive behaviour.

The need for care and support

When clients assault the staff who care for them, the incident is often managed in a way that places emphasis on the client's reaction and behaviour rather than that of the victim. In particular in psychiatric settings, staff will tolerate what are in fact criminal acts, because they recognise that their patients are not responsible and such staff may even blame themselves as responsible professionals for not managing the situation more effectively and thus allowing the assault to occur.

Where the onset of stressful after-effects is delayed, staff find that this is often more difficult to cope with because they have seemed to manage their reaction successfully for a protracted period and cannot explain to themselves their new and perplexing inability to put the incident behind them and to resolve their reaction to it.

Research by Bamber (1992) suggests that properly organised debriefing following the incident can reduce and often prevent the development of more severe and long-term post-traumatic effects. He states that without the opportunity for debriefing, staff tend to react to trauma in two ways:

(a) by isolating themselves, in finding a quiet area in which to unwind
(b) by bottling up the experience and carrying on as if nothing had happened, thus denying any effect.

Engel & Marsh (1986) used a series of follow-up interviews at relevant intervals after an assaultive incident and found that this assisted staff to come to terms with what had happened and allowed them to continue working without further disturbing psychological sequelae. They also suggested that covering up and denying the situation "demoralises front-line workers and negatively affects patient care".

The most effective methods of intervention

Care of assaulted staff requires different levels of intervention at different stages, and how and when it is carried out immediately after the incident depends on the need for physical treatment of the victim. McCloy (1992) suggests that there are three stages of intervention: immediately after the event, short term, and long term. If immediate care is sufficient to allow staff to continue in a satisfactory way with their work then there is no need to intervene in the short or long term. For those who require short-term follow-up care, some will then manage to return to work successfully and will not need the final, long-term intervention, which will then be offered to those who have been more severely traumatised. McCloy's interest is with the fire service, with firemen traumatised when dealing with unpleasant or particularly dramatic incidents, but the principles for the type of staff care that he proposes are effective in all areas of trauma management and equally efficacious with staff who are the victims of assault.

Immediate care

When someone is assaulted, the physical injury needs to be dealt with first. If the injury is slight and does not require hospital admission, the victim should be given peace and quiet in privacy to provide an opportunity for him/her to deal with the immediate emotional reaction. It is then helpful if a senior 'line' manager or someone in a counselling position to the victim spends time in a one-to-one interview to assess the psychological effects of the assault and to allow the victim to talk through perceptions of what happened and how he/she feels about it.

There should be a critical-incident debriefing with all staff present at the incident within 48–72 hours to allow the victim or victims (provided they are physically able and feel that they can cope) to be clear about what actually happened. This aids the victim to process the event cognitively, in order to help make sense out of what is often a confused and confusing picture. Bringing together all those involved allows 'jigsawing' – putting together everyone's small piece of experience to make a coherent and clear picture of the events leading up to, during and immediately after the incident. Everyone, including the victim, is then able to establish their role in the overall incident, which is an important part of beginning to cope with the experience. Critical-incident debriefing involves asking three questions:

(a) What happened?
(b) How did you feel?
(c) How do you feel now?

It also provides an opportunity for peer-group support, and allows people to discuss their reactions together in a way which provides all the group with the reassurance that their emotional reactions are not unusual and that all involved have had similar experiences. As discussed in Chapter 6, it is essential that the debriefing is carried out in a supportive atmosphere.

Bamber (1992) prefers to provide what he terms 'psychological debriefing', which involves similar discussion as critical-incident debriefing but at a more intense level and would require the supervision of a specifically trained senior staff member to lead and facilitate the debriefing. He defines psychological debriefing as "a group meeting arranged for the purposes of integrating profound personal experiences on the cognitive, emotional and group level, thus preventing the development of adverse reactions". He lists seven objectives:

(a) the ventilation of impressions, feelings and reactions
(b) the promotion of cognitive organisation through a clear understanding of events and reactions
(c) decreasing group and individual tension
(d) emphasising the normality of the experience
(e) increasing group support and cohesiveness
(f) preparation for symptoms or reactions which may arise
(g) identifying resources available to help.

It is also very important to give practical information to the victim about the possible after-effects of a stressful experience, providing straightforward advice about how to manage these and help the victim to identify a support system should the need arise for further support. Information should be offered about what to do if these effects persist or increase in intensity, and who to approach should the victim feel that further treatment or support is needed. It is important to ensure that the victim understands that any emotional changes or reactions are those to be expected in anyone exposed to a similarly stressful event. This provides reassurance that this is not the onset of a psychiatric illness, but a normal reaction to an abnormal and aversive experience.

There has been a tendency in public-sector organisations to view providing information to staff about the possible effects of stress as an invitation to staff to 'catch stress' and thus increase absence on sick leave. In my experience this denial has led to higher negative stress levels as staff struggle to cope in ignorance with psychological reactions which frighten them and are intensified by their fear that they are 'having a nervous breakdown'. This macho-style denial approach has largely been broken down in the Scottish Prison Service following the incident-ridden years from 1985 to 1989 and the recognition of the effects of these throughout the Service, but it still persists among some staff and managers within the system. Although debriefing all staff involved occurs as a matter of course, there is also an expectation by staff that their emotional reactions to the incident will be managed in a healthy and positive way. As clinical psychologists working within the system, my colleagues and I offer support to staff following incidents and many staff are quick to use our help. However, there are still some officers who find it difficult to approach us because they fear that having to admit difficulty in coping with their reactions is a personal failure, and that seeking professional help is an acceptance of inadequacy in themselves. McCloy (1992) suggests that within the fire service similar attitudes prevail. Concern that "admissions of stress might prevent promotion" means that peer-group support and advice should be provided at similar-ranking levels, so that fears and emotional reactions can be admitted to without partiality.

If this level of intervention is not wholly successful in managing the immediate emotional reactions caused by the incident, then staff involved may continue to experience difficulties in adjusting and coming to terms with the incident.

Psychological reactions

The most commonly reported difficulties following assaults are a feeling of increased anxiety and threat and thus increased muscle tension, feelings of shock and disbelief, sleep disturbance with nightmares, and intrusive images and thoughts about the incident. Other reactions reported are disturbances of concentration, anger, depression, increased irritability, crying with no reason, a feeling of powerlessness, increased vulnerability, and changes in personal beliefs and value systems. In relation to work, victims report feelings of professional incompetence, a fear of returning to work, phobic reactions to the area of work in which the incident occurred, an expectation of a negative change in their relationship with their colleagues, and, in some cases, feeling sorry for and guilty about the assaultive client. In the longer term, these feelings can develop into burn-out, loss of appetite, physical illnesses such as hypertension and ulcers, increased absenteeism, and performance difficulties; there may also be an increase in the use of alcohol or medication to cope with the stress.

Lanza (1983) suggests that many staff deny experiencing emotional reactions to an assault because she feels that if they admitted their feelings, they would be overwhelmed and it is this process of denial which is responsible for the under-reporting of abusive and assaultive incidents perpetrated by patients in their care.

The following case example illustrates some of the after-effects of an assault on a prison employee:

Case example 7.1

A civilian employee in a prison was assaulted by three prisoners in order to effect an escape. The prisoners had been working 'overtime' for the employee in a workshop in the evenings and he had chosen them to do the work because he considered them good workers and reasonably trustworthy. While he was working, the prisoners had roughly grabbed him from behind and tied him up, one of them apologising throughout for what he was doing and insisting that he meant the instructor no harm. The instructor struggled with the three men and received strain injuries and bruising. Following the incident he reported difficulty in sleeping, with intrusive thoughts about the incident constantly running through his mind and keeping him awake. He said he felt unable to relax or maintain his concentration, even on activities that he enjoyed and normally viewed as ways of providing a contrast to his work and thoughts about it. He became irritable and impatient and difficult to live with. He also described feeling overwhelming panic while waiting to cross the road in town if people came up behind him, which led to him trying to avoid crowded public places. This caused considerable marital friction as his wife enjoyed, and used as a way of managing her stress, the weekend visit by both of them to a busy town for a shopping trip and lunch in the town centre. She found his social withdrawal difficult to understand and manage, and he was unable to explain to her why he was reacting in this way and why he had become so intolerant. The instructor's overriding concern was disappointment that prisoners with whom he had built a good rapport and had trusted to work with him unsupervised in the evenings had betrayed this trust. This led him to suspect his judgement of others and thus his profess–ional skills and confidence, so that going to work became a threat and although, with clinical psychology support and graded exposure to his working environment, he managed the stress-related symptoms such as muscle tension, concentration and sleep difficulties and returned to work after the incident, he lost all enjoyment and satisfaction with his work and eventually took early retirement.

Short-term care

In some areas a consultation service team of peers has been set up for psychiatric nursing staff who are victims of assault (Engel & Marsh, 1986; Murray & Snyder, 1991; Flannery *et al*, 1991) to good effect. Murray & Snyder found an enthusiastic response to their nursing consultation service, which they felt highlighted the need for a supportive, non-blaming response to the assaulted staff victim and reinforced the importance of acknowledging emotional conse-quences of assault in the health care field. The consultation teams see the victim one to four times, providing the opportunity to describe the incident in detail, to look at what caused it and what happened as a result. The consultation group member works with the victim in looking at the emotional reactions to the incident and also at the attribution of blame. The service provides a problem-solving approach to facilitate learning of positive coping strategies in both the management and the prevention of future incidents.

Engel & Marsh (1986) described the establishment of a hospital policy to care for physically abused staff which stated that "employees who are subject to physical attacks are to be given high priority with regard to medical and psychosocial care". The policy mandated immediate medical and emotional care, legal and practical advice, follow-up treatment, psychosocial counselling for employees, and a well timed investigation of the incident and documentation of the incident and injury.

Flannery *et al* (1991) describe the Voluntary Assaulted Staff Action Programme, set up in 1990 to offer support to staff victims of patient violence in a state mental hospital. They found that traumatised victims who are given the opportunity to discuss the traumatic incident immediately after it occurs often cope more effectively, without any disturbing after-effects. They state that keeping reasonable control in the work situation, having a caring support system and the ability to make some sense of the event are significant factors affecting post-traumatic adaptation. The programme team is made up of 15 volunteer clinicians from all disciplines, who are each on call via a bleeper system for a period of 24 hours. These line staff have rostered supervisors who are also held on call and who then provide critical-incident debriefing to wards on which a distressing incident has occurred. This involves a review of the event, an update on the health of the victim, and a focus on the thoughts, affects and symptoms that the victim might be experiencing, closing with suggestions for coping more adaptively. Short-term weekly support groups are provided for victims, and the programme team can arrange meetings for victims' families to aid them in understanding and adjusting to the emotional impact of the assault. The team also offers support to colleagues of the victim, with the aim of reducing the level of general stress on the wards and thus indirectly helping to prevent future assaults.

Longer-term care

If symptoms persist or increase in severity it is important that professional help be sought, as the victim may suffer post-traumatic stress disorder (PTSD). Caldwell (1992) used questionnaires with two groups of mental health staff to attempt to establish the incidence of assault and resulting symptoms of PTSD among them. He reports that 52% of those returning the questionnaire had some symptoms of, and 9% warranted a diagnosis of, PTSD. In spite of frequent traumatic events in the working environments of these staff, he reports that organisational support for traumatised staff was minimal or non-existent.

Symptoms of PTSD

The American Psychiatric Association (DSM–IV; 1994) defines the essential feature of PTSD (309.81) in adults as being "the development of characteristic symptoms

(a) following exposure to an extreme traumatic stressor involving:
  (i)   direct personal experience of an event that involves actual or threatened death or serious injury, or other threat to one's physical integrity; or witnessing an event that involves death, injury or a threat to the physical integrity of another person; or learning about unexpected or violent death, serious harm, or threat of death or injury experienced by a family member or other close associate.
  (ii)   a personal response to the stressor involving intense fear, helplessness or horror.
(b) the traumatic event is persistently re-experienced in one or more of the following ways:
  (i)   recurrent and intrusive distressing recollections of the event, including images, thoughts or perceptions
  (ii)   recurrent distressing dreams of the event
  (iii) acting or feeling as if the traumatic event were recurring (includes a sense of reliving the experience, illusions, hallucinations and dissociative flashback episodes, including those that occur on awakening or when intoxicated)
  (iv)   intense psychological distress at exposure to internal or external cues that symbolise or resemble an aspect of the traumatic event
  (v)   physiological reactivity on exposure to internal or external cues that symbolise or resemble an aspect of the traumatic event.
(c) persistent avoidance of stimuli associated with the trauma and numbing of general responsiveness (not present before the trauma), as indicated by three (or more) of the following:
  (i)   efforts to avoid thoughts, feelings or conversations associated with the trauma
  (ii)   efforts to avoid activities, places, or people that arouse recollections of the trauma
  (iii) inability to recall an important aspect of the trauma
  (iv)   markedly diminished interest or participation in significant activities
  (v)   feeling of detachment or estrangement from others

- (vi) restricted range of affect (e.g. unable to have loving feelings
- (vii) sense of foreshortened future (e.g. does not expect to have a career, marriage, children, or a normal life span).
- (d) persistent symptoms of increased arousal (not present before the trauma), as indicated by two (or more) of the following:
  - (i) difficulty falling or staying asleep
  - (ii) irritability or outbursts or anger
  - (iii) difficulty concentrating
  - (iv) hypervigilance
  - (v) exaggerated startle response
- (e) duration of the disturbance (symptoms in criteria b, c, and d) is more than one month
- (f) the disturbance causes clinically significant distress or impairment in social, occupational, or other important areas of functioning.

Acute PTSD: duration of symptoms less than three months
Chronic PTSD: duration of symptoms is three months or more
PTSD with delayed onset: if onset of symptoms is at least six months after stressor".

If PTSD develops, then professional psychological or psychiatric support should be sought.

Who should provide the care?

At the immediate stage, as discussed earlier, initial debriefing should be carried out on site by the line manager or supervisor of the area, or by a member of staff trained and available for such a purpose. Simple information packs listing possible after-effects and how to manage them, where to go for support, and what to do if symptoms persist and intensify should be provided not just to the direct victims but to all staff involved in an incident. On-lookers, particularly those close to the victim, can also be traumatised quite dramatically. Guilt at one's impotence to save the victim or prevent the assault is common, particularly for those close to the victim. In any close-knit working team, responsibility for what happens during the working day is shared by all members of that team; this offers positive support but can also result in shared attribution of self-blame and trauma.

The short-term stage should be managed by line managers and primary health care, that is, a general practitioner and the occupational health service, but if the problem intensifies or becomes long-term, then it is important that clinical psychology or psychiatric support be offered.

Summary of procedures for the management of staff who are assaulted in their workplace

(a) Physical care must be provided for injuries, and privacy arranged to allow the victim to come to terms with the immediate emotional reaction.

(b) A structured and focused debriefing 48–72 hours after the incident should be managed by a competent and trained member of staff, to allow all staff involved to ventilate and to piece together what actually happened. Staff should be encouraged to examine and acknowledge their emotional reactions and to offer each other support to manage similar incidents more effectively. The normality and communality of the emotional reaction should be emphasised, and information given on possible further reactions and how to manage these. It is useful to provide simple information packs on this and on the resources available for support should the need arise. Immediately after an incident, many people may not be able to remember information accurately, however important.

(c) Staff victims of assault should be provided with a written summary of their rights and how to apply for compensation.

(d) Follow-up of staff continuing to be traumatised by the assault after the debriefing should be arranged, and this should be carried out in an interview with a line manager or trained colleague. For those who continue to have difficulties, further contact should be arranged to monitor progress and to offer referral to the occupational health service or to the victim's general practitioner. It is helpful if a specifically designated and appropriately trained member of staff carries out the follow-up and that management are aware of the special nature of the needs of assaulted staff. Welfare difficulties should also be assessed and managed, and victims should not be left to wade through the frustrations of bureaucracy unaided.

(e) If distressing emotional reactions continue and intensify, persisting for a period of more than four weeks, it may be that the victim is developing a significant post-traumatic stress reaction and is in need of further referral to a clinical psychologist or a psychiatrist.

Factors affecting reactions to an incident

Why do some people cope effectively – what are effective coping strategies?

Stress is incremental, so the level of stress that a person is carrying before the assault happens is important. If a member of staff has experienced a major life event or is feeling vulnerable and is questioning his/her professional skills and motivation before an incident, an assault can provide the 'final straw' in terms of confirming any negative ideas associated with work or life in general. If victims are able to make sense of what happened to them and see the assault as a one-off event, stimulated by specific and controllable triggers (see Chapter 4), it is easier to accept and to plan future prevention. Constructive and positive reactions enable victims to reassert control over their environment and to regain confidence in their professional skills. Successful management of such a stressor may even contribute to personal development, strengthening confidence and providing reassurance that one is able to overcome even the most feared of adversity.

The ability to re-establish beliefs in one's own security at work and the understanding of how and why the incident occurred are crucial in the recovery process, because they allow the victim to discriminate between a one-off problem and a constant threat, and they promote the belief that such an incident is unlikely to occur again or on a regular basis. The victim can then rehearse positive ways of preventing recurrence and can adopt strategies that allow reconstruction and strengthening of the view that one is prepared to cope with any further difficulties. If victims do not perceive the experience in this way and retain the feeling that they are constantly under threat, demotivation will prevent effective functioning at work.

What are the environmental and organisational influences on reactions to incidents?

On the assumption that a good management team values well trained and experienced staff who work effectively, management's aim will be to handle the after-effects of a serious and assaultive incident in a way which will reinforce confidence in their concern for their staff and their commitment to providing a working environment that is secure and supportive.

It is vitally important that management is seen to be interested in staff wellbeing and safety. Good management during a crisis can increase team cohesion and protect staff by supporting them in coping effectively with difficult and unpredictable clients. Reduction of environmental and occupational stressors can provide predictability in a working situation so that the only unpredictable factor is client behaviour, thus keeping day-to-day stressors to a minimum. Frustration becomes apparent if staff have continually informed management about potential risk areas or activities and dangers but no clear action has been taken – this adds to the anger and hostility felt by victims and increases fear of return to work.

It is important that assaulted staff are given support and information about compensation, demonstrating that management are concerned about welfare; petty wrangles about money further alienate staff who lose confidence in management or feel that they were assaulted because their employers had failed to take precautions against such an incident. Legal help for a compensation claim is provided free by many trade unions and some professional organisations.

Case example 7.2

A prison officer who had been taken hostage was subsequently faced by his finance department's refusal to recognise the time (over 20 hours) he had spent being held hostage as working time. While the people close to him were attempting to help him re-establish his identity as a professional prison officer, a distant but powerful civil servant was implying that by being taken hostage he ceased to be a valued professional employee of the organisation at work, deserving of remuneration for that work. Happily the organisation has learned from such early mistakes – an identified line manager now carries out all discussion with the pay office and human resources department so that the individual does not have to deal with such matters directly.

Sometimes staff who come to terms quickly and effectively with the experience of being assaulted find that they are not allowed to put their experience behind them in a natural way because sympathetic colleagues constantly enquire in a significant way about their welfare long after the event. This interferes with the process of the assaulted person throwing off the role of victim and reassuming the more positive role of responsible professional member of staff.

For many staff it helps to get back to the situation in which they were assaulted as soon as possible – the analogy is with falling off a horse and remounting immediately to reduce the fear of riding again. This allows victims to reassert their professional status and to reassure themselves that they can cope. Management can play an important role in offering flexible working hours and practice for victims in order to allow them to reintegrate at their own pace. The outcome of this flexibility often costs fewer man-hours than adhering to a 'set shift pattern or nothing' ruling, which can force staff on to sick leave because they are not immediately able to cope with full-time responsibilities in a potentially threatening environment without a graded re-exposure. It takes time to rebuild confidence and comfort in an environment which has traumatised them.

Managers, particularly those of areas in which staff assaults are likely to occur, should receive training in the needs of traumatised staff so that they can develop well informed and best-practice procedures to deal with the problem in their working areas.

What are the personal factors which influence victims' reactions?

Good peer-group support is extremely important and staff who have a wide-ranging group of friends among their workmates and who can use them to good effect tend to cope better than staff who are socially isolated among their peers. The level and success of a social-support system plays a complex part in recovery, as found in a study by Whittington & Wykes (1992). The support in this study was provided informally at three interviews and was concentrated on the period immediately following the incident. Levels of strain were measured using the Spielberger Self-evaluation Questionnaire and a questionnaire designed by the authors based on items suggested by a review of the literature on the effects of trauma. The results suggested that high levels of strain are associated with high levels of support, but discussion of this purely preliminary study suggested that the support was provided only on a very short-term informal basis, so that there was no formal longer-term system for providing staff with proper opportunities to come to terms with their experience. The implication is that no matter how good and caring a personal support system is, managing the after-effects of a traumatic assault must be carried out in a structured, informed and professional way.

The presence of other stressors, such as marital or relationship difficulties, financial problems or lack of physical fitness, previous experience of an assault, and the degree to which one's personal view of the world is disrupted also contribute to the way in which a victim copes with an assault. Premorbid personality factors and existing problems such as depression and generalised anxiety predispose victims to cope less effectively with traumatic stressors and increase the impact of the traumatic event.

The choice of date for return to work after the incident is very important; an assaulted member of staff needs time and space to recover equilibrium, but often the longer the absence, the more difficult going back to work becomes; equally, returning to work too early and failing to cope reinforces the role of victim and delays the recovery of professional confidence, and may thus lead to longer absenteeism. A member of staff who appears to cope well initially with an assault may, as a result of further life stressors such as a bereavement, breakdown of a close relationship or further aggressive incidents at work, even only of a verbal type, find that contingent on these, there are emotional difficulties in coping with the original incident, such as 'flashbacks' and intrusive thoughts and images not previously not experienced.

Differential individual coping strategies create differences in coming to terms with experiences, and the repertoire of skills that staff carry to deal with stressors will determine the way in which they will deal with their emotional reaction to the incident.

What is the role of violence in staff burn-out?

Emotional reactions to traumatic assaults will, if not managed properly, lead to burn-out. If post-traumatic effects such as hyper-vigilance, hypervulnerability and emotional blunting occur, then it is difficult to maintain the motivation to continue working and personal effectiveness is diminished. Badly apportioned blame can leave staff feeling that they are no longer fit for their job or have no wish to continue in a job which can expose an employee to such an aversive experience. Lack of confidence in management to provide a safe environment for their staff or anger at the way in which staff are managed following an aggressive incident with a client also leads to demotivation, poor morale and a loss of job satisfaction.

Returning to work is especially difficult for staff taken hostage: "the penalty for a live hostage is often a hostile hostage" (Bolz, 1979). Where staff are taken hostage by a client, their role as carers or custodians is dramatically shattered and their lack of control over their situation sudden and profound. During the negotiation process hostages feel isolated from their professional peers and abandoned by the organisation for which they work. Hostages are often forced into a relationship with their captor by this feeling and by the need to relate on a personal level with the person who appears to directly control their safety and destiny. The instinctive formation of a close positive relationship with the perpetrator can make it more difficult for the perpetrator to damage the hostage and thus provides protection. Management of hostage incidents can often lead to the hostage apparently being discounted, as the authorities (often the hostage's own employers) take their time in bargaining the fate of the hostage. The perception of the hostage is sometimes that it is the perpetrator who appears to be more genuinely and directly interested in the hostage's welfare and that the authorities appear to be resisting the perpetrator's attempts to end the incident quickly and without injury (see Chapter 4 for further discussion of hostage incidents). The anger and resentment experienced during the incident towards the authorities persists long after the incident is over if the hostage is not properly debriefed and cared for, and builds into a communication barrier even with a well motivated management honestly and sympathetically trying to reintegrate the member of staff into a working environment, whether it is the one in which they were taken hostage or a carefully chosen client-free new one. The motivation to continue working for what is perceived to be such a bad employer is poor and may lead to resignation of an experienced and valued staff member or requests for transfer to a less threatening workplace.

Hostage taking is the extreme end of a staff assault continuum, but any level of assault produces similar reactions to poor management and care of victims. If management places emphasis on the care of an assaultive patient, while forgetting the assaulted staff member, the victim is left feeling resentful and isolated.

Equally, failure on the part of an employer to recognise that recovery of a victim can take considerable time can lead to frustration that the victim seems to be unwilling to cooperate with what management perceive as generous and patient attempts to offer suitable working environments following the incident.

How do colleagues react and how should this be managed?

For many staff who are victims of assault by their clients the attitude of some of their colleagues who make critical and hurtful remarks is a real and damaging problem.

Some staff shun their colleagues who have been assaulted, almost as if assault might be 'catching', because there is a need to see the victim as different and possibly less capable than oneself in order to maintain one's own perception that assault happens to others. This allows such staff to maintain as sacrosanct their belief that they are intrinsically safe, even though they work in the same environment as the victim with the same violent clients. (Among certain prison staff there is an expectation that after being assaulted they are entitled to some time off on sick leave, and such staff view with hostility those who return to work immediately after an assault.)

Great interest, sympathy and support are shown by colleagues to the victim initially, but this eventually dies a natural death, and then can come the 'should have pulled himself together by now' attitude by staff towards a colleague who continues to have difficulty in coming to terms with an experience, beyond the period that peers consider acceptable. There is an analogy with people's reaction to bereavement and the way in which, once the immediate fuss and concern has died down, the bereaved person is faced suddenly with the full impact of the loss and sudden loneliness in the need to cope alone without support.

In working with staff held hostage and observing the reactions of their colleagues and managers there still seems to be difficulty in recognising that the experience of being held hostage can have life-shattering effects and that the victim's personal belief system can be changed for life and that the victim will react differently for several years.

Case example 7.3

Managers discussed a nurse who had been held hostage some five years previously; she had been inadequately supported after the incident. The suggestion was made that the woman was 'putting on' doubts and fears about her work 'just to get sympathy' and, out of 'laziness', to avoid duty in the situation in which she had been taken hostage. The nurse continued to have nightmares and flashbacks about the incident, and the working situation into which it was proposed to move her had significant elements of the environment in which the incident had taken place; these elements could trigger further flashbacks and interfere with her ability to carry out this work.

Professional treatment

The following techniques have been used to manage the post-traumatic reactions of victims of assault:

'Ventilation' and supportive counselling

This comprises the opportunity to talk freely about the victim's perceptions of the assaultive experience both factually and emotionally, with the support of the therapist to explain and clarify the emotional reactions and actions of the victim and others involved in the experience.

Cognitive–behavioural therapy

People experience and react to incidents on the basis of their individual personal perception of the occurrence and their views of how competent they are to manage it. The internal dialogue that all of us use to mediate our experiences and incorporate them into our belief system determines our reactions to any stimulus, and the personal belief system or framework against which we measure our world is created from such past experience and learning. Disruption of this framework and the inability to assimilate a crisis satisfactorily causes dysfunctioning of the internal dialogue.

The cognitive–behavioural approach seeks to examine the dialogue, identify dysfunctional and negative thoughts, and provide alternative positive self-talk to improve functioning. This allows re-establishment of the personal framework and constructs in such a way as to improve coping skills, providing confidence to return to a working environment initially viewed as threatening.

An example of this approach is as follows. A nurse in the long-stay ward in which she normally works views her work area as a place in which she is safe and in control. Her internal dialogue reflects this belief and is made up of self-statements such as "I know how to cope when I'm in my own patch", "the patients I work with know and respect me and wouldn't dream of harming me", "If I manage a confrontation with skill then I won't be hurt". An assault on the nurse by one of her patients immediately throws all these statements into question, and unless she is able restate her belief about her security in a positive way by modifying her self-talk to accept that such an event can happen, but that she is equipped to deal with it, she will find it extremely difficult to return to her workplace. Cognitive restructuring will help her form positive coping self-statements, such as "my work area is safe provided I don't make assumptions about my patients' behaviour", "I can recognise potential confrontation and act to prevent it", "Incidents do happen but they are infrequent and there is always a reason for them, by assessing potential difficulties and using problem-solving to resolve them, I can make my workplace safer".

Stress inoculation training

This is designed to build 'psychological antibodies', or coping skills, and to enhance resistance through exposure to stimuli that are strong enough to arouse defences without being so powerful as to overcome them (Meichenbaum, 1985). Stress inoculation is like providing patients with credits for stress management; these credits are used whenever they are faced with traumatic situations: coping well gains more credit by confirming skills, but coping badly uses up the credits provided or gained, and old skills need to be practised or replaced by more effective ones.

There are three phases to stress inoculation training:

(a) the conceptualisation phase, in which rapport is established, information about the stressful event and the victim's emotional reactions to it collated, and a reconceptualisation of the victim's stress reactions provided
(b) the skills acquisition and rehearsal phase, in which the victim is helped to develop and consolidate a variety of coping strategies, which emerge naturally from the first phase; training techniques used include relaxation training, cognitive restructuring, problem solving and self-instructional training (this training needs to be individually tailored to the victim's needs)
(c) the application and follow-through phase, in which the victim rehearses coping skills in training sessions and in real situations; possible methods include imagery and behavioural rehearsal, modelling, role play, and graduated exposure. Relapse prevention and follow-up also form part of this phase.

Prolonged exposure

This is a technique which involves reliving the traumatising incident in imagination – imaginal exposure. Patients are asked to talk through their experience in the present tense and are encouraged to imagine the scene as vividly as possible ('as if you are there') and they are required to relive the scenario as many times as possible during a one-hour session. Recordings of the sessions are given as homework to patients, who are asked to listen to them at least once a day between sessions. Other homework involves real-life exposure to feared and avoided trigger situations as judged appropriate by patient and therapist.

Systematic desensitisation and graded exposure

These are methods of working through situations of incrementally increasing trauma by imaginal exposure (desensitisation) and real-life practice (graded exposure). The patient prepares a hierarchy of situations which arouse varying degrees of stress, from least to most, and then, following relaxation training, imagines the first, least anxiety-provoking scene while relaxed, practising until the scene can be relived without any increase in tension. Having achieved total relaxation with this situation, the patient repeats the procedure with each increasingly stressful scene until the hierarchy has been worked through. Once a trigger situation has been successfully dealt with in imagination, practice is transferred to the real-life situation in graded exposure, continuing to use relaxation techniques to control physical tension.

Case example 7.4

This technique was used successfully with a prison officer who had been taken hostage. Following the use of systematic desensitisation on a hierarchy of increasingly stressful work situations, he returned to work in the prison in a post which had limited prisoner contact. In this post he did not need to enter the prison halls, one of which had been the scene of the hostage taking. In conjunction with his line manager, the clinical psychologist arranged that he move to tasks involving increasing prisoner contact. He remained in each new working situation until he could cope to his satisfaction without increased physiological arousal or a wish to avoid the task. He then spent some time in each of the prison halls, firstly when prisoners were out of the hall at work or locked up in cell, and then in increasingly crowded times of day with prisoners circulating in the hall. Gradually he coped successfully with increasingly stressful areas until he was able to return to work in the feared hall with little negative emotional reaction, finding that with the successful completion of each incremental task, his confidence to move forwards was increased.

Desensitisation differs from prolonged exposure in that imaginal exposure is used while the patient is relaxed, whereas in the prolonged exposure technique the patient is not relaxed but is encouraged to re-experience anxiety as strongly as possible.

Relaxation techniques

The provision of training in muscular relaxation techniques allows the victim to reassert physical control and provides a simple way of managing psychophysiological symptoms such as hyperventilation, panic, insomnia, and muscle tension.

Hypnosis

Hypnosis can also be used to achieve deep muscular relaxation, but in addition provides the opportunity to use positive self-suggestion to combat negative and intrusive thinking. Mental rehearsal of successful management of the traumatising incident during hypnotic trance can provide positive exposure to the feared situation, re-establishing self-confidence.

Foa *et al* (1991) conducted a survey into the comparative effectiveness of different therapeutic approaches in the treatment of rape victims suffering from PTSD. Using a waiting-list control group, they compared prolonged imaginal exposure to the rape trauma, stress inoculation training and supportive counselling. Supportive counselling was included to control for possible therapist effects. They found that stress inoculation training was most effective in reducing

Summary points

- There should be clear guidelines and standard operating procedures for the management of violent incidents and the emotional reactions of the staff involved in them. Good practice requires knowledge and training about the processes and reactions involved and how to manage these effectively, so that staff do not develop PTSD, and are not lost as a result of demotivation and burn-out. Clinical psychologists can provide effective training to managers and volunteers to prevent the development of maladaptive reactions and behaviours which would otherwise follow assaultive incidents.
- Workplace assaults on staff in the caring professions can be particularly distressing to victims because it may challenge their sense of role, and their confidence in their professional skills.
- Staff may suppress their response to an incident and, in some cases, the reaction can be delayed. Organisations should make plans for immediate, short-term and long-term support, adapted to a victim's requirements.
- Immediate support should include a carefully run debriefing session for all those involved. Victims should be given information on possible reactions to the event, and advice on how to obtain further help. Providing information does not make staff more likely to experience reactions.
- PTSD is uncommon but serious, and requires careful clinical management.
- Hostage episodes can be very distressing for the victim, who may feel abandoned. Advance training and post-incident support can be of great assistance in minimising distress.
- The organisation has to ensure that a comprehensive support system is in place, and that victims are helped with financial and administrative problems resulting from the incident. There should be flexibility in time-tabling and allocation of duties following an incident.
- A variety of psychological techniques can be used to help victims. It is important to adapt choice of technique to the circumstances of the incident and the needs of the individual staff member.

symptoms immediately after treatment, but that three and a half months after treatment finished prolonged exposure appeared to be the most effective treatment. Patients treated with supportive counselling or left on the waiting-list seemed to show improvement in the management of arousal symptoms of PTSD but not of intrusion and avoidance symptoms. They explained their findings by the fact that the prolonged exposure technique is thought to lead to permanent change in the memory of the trauma, and hence to durable gains, whereas stress inoculation training uses anxiety management, which provides mainly immediate relief. They state that exposure treatments facilitate the emotional processing of the memory of the incident, including habituation to feared stimuli, re-evaluation of the probability of threat in feared situations, and changes in the negative 'valence' associated with fear responses. They also consider that real-life exposure is an important ingredient in the reduction of avoidance in anxiety-disordered individuals. Their work demonstrated that depression and anxiety decreased significantly following all treatments, including the waiting-list group, suggesting that mere contact with a therapist is sufficient to reduce general distress although not specific PTSD symptoms. The authors suggest that combining stress inoculation techniques with prolonged exposure might provide a more comprehensively effective approach, and that this should form the basis for future research.

A model of treatment

From my own experience of treating victims of assault and hostage taking, it is important to use elements of several techniques at different stages throughout therapy and to tailor treatment to patient needs. The assessment of what elements of what therapeutic approach are needed is made on the basis of my clinical experience, monitoring of the patient's response, and patient preference and ability to manage the concept involved. These techniques should be as useful in health care or social work settings as they are in prisons.

Once the patient has had the opportunity to ventilate feelings, it is important to develop a clear, chronologically accurate description of the incident, and working towards this allows exposure to the memory of the assault. Access to official logs or accounts of the incident are useful for clarifying events. After any incident, prison officers are asked to write a paper describing exactly what they perceived as happening, and these offer useful information on distorted memories and perceptions for the victim.

I offer simple relaxation training at the first session to provide immediate relief of many of the physical symptoms of PTSD; it is also an important first step in demonstrating to patients that it is possible for them to begin to reassert control. Using the final detailed description of the incident we then work through the emotional experiences associated with the event, and from there look at the cognitive elements occurring before, during, and after the assault. It is important that patients can recognise the changes in self-talk and in their belief system so that we can then work towards rebuilding and reprocessing these to provide a more effective personal framework and coping strategies.

Further research on the effectiveness of specific elements of therapeutic interventions for specific elements of PTSD is required, particularly in relation to the type of trauma undergone, premorbid factors and future targets in relation to coping at work following an assault by a client.

References

AMERICAN PSYCHIATRIC ASSOCIATION (1994) *Diagnostic and Statistical Manual of Mental Disorders* (4th edn) (DSM–IV). WASHINGTON DC: APA.

BAMBER, M. (1992) Debriefing victims of violence. *Occupational Health*, April,115–117.

BOLZ, F. (1983) The hostage situation: law enforcement options. In *Terrorism: Interdisciplinary Perspectives* (eds B. Eichelman, D. Soskis & W. Reid). Washington DC: APA.

CALDWELL, M. F. (1992) Incidence of PTSD among staff victims of patient violence. *Hospital and Community Psychiatry*, **43**, 838–839.

CONN, L. M. & LION, J. R. (1983) Assault in a university hospital. In *Assault within Psychiatric Facilities* (eds J. R. Lion & W. H. Reid). pp 61–69. New York: Grune & Stratton.

ENGEL, F. & MARSH, S. (1986) Helping the employee victim of violence in hospitals. *Hospital and Community Psychiatry*, **37**, 159–162.

FLANNERY, R. B. JR., FULTON, P., TAUSCH, J., et al (1991) A program to help staff cope with psychological sequelae of assaults by patients. *Hospital and Community Psychiatry*, **42**, 935–938.

FOA, E. B., ROTHBAUM, B. C., RIGGS, D. S., et al (1991) Treatment of post-traumatic stress disorder in rape victims: a comparison between cognitive-behavioural procedures and councelleing. *Journal of Consulting and Clinical Psychology*, **59**, 715–723.

JANOFF-BULMAN, R. & FRIEZE, R. (1983) A theoretical perspective for understanding reactions to victimisation. *Journal of Social Issues*, **39**, 1-17.

LANZA, M. L. (1983) the reactions of nursing staff to physical assault by a patient. *Hospital and Community Psychiatry*, **34**, 44–47.

—— (1985) Counselling services for staff victims of patient assault. *Administration in Mental Health*, **12**, 205–207.

McCLOY, E. (1992) Management of post-incident trauma: a fire service perspective. *Occupational Medicine*, **42**, 163–166.

MEICHENBAUM, D. (1985) *Stress Inoculation Training*. Oxford: Pergamon Press.

MURRAY, M. G. & SNYDER, J. C. (1991) When staff are assaulted. A nursing consultation support service. *Journal of Psychosocial Nursing and Mental Health Services*, **29**, 24–29.

POSTER, E. C. & RYAN, J. A. (1989) Nurses' attitudes towards physical assaults by patients. *Archives of Psychiatric Nursing*, **3**, 315–322.

RYAN, J. A. & POSTER, E. C. (1989) The assaulted nurse: short-term and long-term responses. *Archives of Psychiatric Nursing*, **3**, 323–331.

WHITTINGTON, R. & WYKES, T. (1992) Staff strain and social support in a psychiatric hospital following assault by a patient. *Journal of Advances in Nursing*, **17**, 480–486.

8 Practical ethical and legal aspects of caring for the assaultive client

FRANCES AIKEN and PAUL TARBUCK

The therapeutic encounter, whether it be in the community, hospital or residential setting, should be a privileged and enjoyable experience for the carer. The client will divulge confidences and innermost thoughts and feelings to the carer about extremely intimate issues and, on occasion, life-threatening experiences; and the carer has the opportunity to focus exclusively upon the needs of another human being and to bring the skills and knowledge associated with a socially respected professional group to the encounter.

Health-care professionals are well aware that as the therapeutic encounter develops the client becomes vulnerable as he/she, for a time, becomes reliant and dependent upon the carer – and because of this may become less able to consider objectively his/her situation and more susceptible to exploitation as a result. The carers themselves are not immune to the uncertainties of their humanity and so the relationship is set within a framework of ethical and legal indicators that characterise the parameters of what is acceptable in this type of human encounter.

The therapeutic encounter is reliant for its success upon the informed consent of the client and within this relationship both the carer and the recipient have roles and responsibilities. In the majority of therapeutic encounters the relationship is beneficial to the client, and the carer finds fulfilment in the therapist's role; however, carers do occasionally find themselves offering assistance to clients who are in great distress or crisis – physically or psychologically; or who do not see the need for the therapeutic relationship and are therefore non-compliant with the prescribed therapy. In these instances clients may become overassertive, angry, aggressive or violent towards the carer, and the ethical and legal parameters of the encounter acquire an added significance – that of providing the client, carer and society with a framework against which actions may be reviewed for their acceptability to all parties, should that become necessary.

This chapter concerns the ethical and legal aspects of the therapeutic encounter that may become foremost when care is being given to the aggressive or potentially violent client, and it is the intention of the writers to consider, and offer guidance upon, some of the dilemmas that health-care professionals face in difficult situations, and readers are asked to reflect upon their own clinical practice in light of the following discussion.

Caring for the client while protecting others from possible aggression

In our everyday lives we are rarely faced with violence or aggression except in the fantasy world of the cinema or at a remote level when we watch the television news. These encounters are by choice – yet as health carers in the field of mental health where the client may be confused, paranoid or hostile we must recognise our moral commitment to care for people who may, at times, be verbally or physically aggressive to us, to their families, the public or other clients. The question is, do we care for them using the most moral interventions possible or do we give custodial care by means of practices that merely contain them or even harm their rights to self-determination, respect and the least restrictive environment possible?

The premise that if we recognise that all clients have rights then we as carers have an obligation to care for them is based on the principle of beneficence, or duty to care, to do good, and the principle of non-maleficence (to prevent harm). These ethical principles are enshrined in the Hippocratic oath and other professional codes of conduct. The paternalistic beneficence that is the hallmark of medical interventions for the mentally ill has been challenged by liberalists who see a conflict between paternalism and respect for the individual's autonomy, insisting that a right of self-determination overrides all other principles:

> "Paternalism in health and social service personnel can lead to the denial of autonomy they should be seeking to promote." (Atkinson, 1991)

Case example 8.1

Freda, a 63-year-old lady, has been on the acute admission ward for six weeks as a formal patient. She has had to have close observation for most of that time as she has expressed ideas of killing herself or others, has been violent at times and is severely depressed. Antidepressants have had no effect and her consultant has now recommended a course of electroconvulsive therapy (ECT), which she refuses to accept. The multidisciplinary team have discussed this: some believe that any intervention is justified as she has been so demanding of resources, with no prospect of improvement, while her primary nurse feels that she is rational enough to understand the information she has been given and the choices open to her. The primary nurse believes that to give her ECT, with no guarantee of benefit, against her wishes, can only harm the therapeutic relationship and her right to self-determination.

The primary nurse believed that Freda's autonomy could be respected while others saw that medical intervention was essential. The paternalistic attitudes of the team seem justified, but their expertise was challenged by the primary nurse's own beliefs in Freda's autonomy.

Unchecked paternalism (however we try to justify it by reasons of acting in the client's 'best interests') may lead to the individual's personality being changed in subtle ways or towards learned helplessness and institutionalisation. Respect for the client's self-determination, alternatively, may result in independence, with rejection of the health carer and services, including medication. This risk may be seen by some mental health practitioners as a threat to their status and authority, and where the client behaves in an antisocial manner a possible danger to the community at large.

We, as practitioners with duties and obligations, are then in the dilemma of either taking risks by respecting autonomy, or controlling the client through interventions such as medication in order to prevent possible future harm. However, the dilemma is not even as straightforward as that. Do we, as public employees, also have to try to impart the most benefit to the greater number of people (utilitarianism) rather than one individual, our client, and thus take into account the wishes of the public? With the current backlash of media attention against the mentally ill should we, then, have to contain clients who have been mentally ill, but do not need hospital admission, longer than that individual actually requires in order to safeguard the public from any risk, no matter how small?

In the microcosm of a psychiatric ward, the dilemma for the professional when managing assaultive clients is still whether to control those most potentially violent and thus protect other clients from harm while decreasing that person's autonomy, or to take a calculated risk to give the individual more freedom and choice. Paternalistic interventions are called for when there is an immediate and obvious risk of harm to others, but these must be tempered with the notions of restoring autonomy as soon as possible, while at the same time working to create more possibilities for autonomy through allowing appropriate decision making, informing the individual who is violent or aggressive of the reasons for temporary control, and by allowing therapeutic interventions to restore to the individual the psychological wherewithal to understand and make the appropriate choices necessary for responsible self-determination.

As carers, do we act as agents of the public, or with the intention of creating individual autonomy?

Case example 8.2

James, a patient on an acute psychiatric ward, became angry that he had received no visits from his relatives for two weeks. He became more suspicious about the staff, accusing them of preventing the visitors seeing him and finally attempting, during visiting time, to hit the staff nurse and a student nurse with a chair. Despite attempts to de-escalate the situation verbally and calm him, James punched the staff nurse, at the same time pushing another patient's visitor out of the way. Other staff who knew James came to the ward and controlled him using approved restraint holds. He was taken to a quiet area, where his primary nurse explained what was happening and gave him the options if he continued his behaviour. James, after ten minutes, consented to stop fighting, was released and talked through the incident with his primary nurse, who offered to ring his relatives for him if he wished.

James's autonomy was curtailed while he was harming others, but the staff attempted to create more autonomy through imparting to him understanding and allowing choices as long as others were not harmed by those choices:

" A very strong reason (although not abiding in all cases) not to respect individual autonomy is when the autonomous decision of the individual will harm one or more other people. Beyond this, the issues must be resolved by personal judgement and compre-hensive and appropriate moral reasoning." (Seedhouse, 1989)

If we cite dangerousness or risk management as a justification for coercive treatment of an assaultive client, we must be extremely cautious that this is valid and that expediency is not a more honest reason when, in a busy ward, medication may be used to tranquillise clients to free staff to undertake other tasks rather than dealing with the demands of this client group.

When at all possible, negotiation with the care team and mutually agreed goals for care, along with explicit informed consent by the client, will reduce the chances of assaultive behaviour:

> "The importance of therapeutic alliance with patients is unquestioned, as is its ethical counterpart, voluntary informed consent." (Eth & Mills, 1990)

To obtain true informed consent from a client who may be unpredictable or thought disordered can be difficult, requiring patience, repeated explanations at the level the patient will understand, and constant checking for understanding as well as agreement. Without this there is a risk of coercion when the professional, who has more power in the relationship, could ignore the client's rights to safety, dignity and freedom from harm; for example, secluding a client for verbal aggression when there is no immediate risk of physical harm and other, more appropriate interventions such as verbal de-escalation have not been attempted. When it has been decided by the care team that a client is incapable of giving informed consent to therapeutic interventions and there is a risk of harm to others, who will make decisions on behalf of that client? Advocacy for vulnerable clients is a contentious issue, as there are risks in assuming the role of advocate. For example, if the advocate has different values from the client he/she may not always act in the way the client would wish. Or, if the advocate is an employee of the organisation that is containing/treating the client, he/she may not be totally objective. However, advocacy is a role that is often forced upon the practitioner in such instances as tranquillising a client who is verbally abusive – a primary nurse may be called upon to act as an advocate on behalf of the client when over-medication interferes with other therapeutic interventions and may be potentially harmful to the therapeutic relationship.

These debates, over the dilemma of possible harm versus respect for autonomy and the demand by the public for security versus the need for therapeutic interventions, continuously arise in the professional literature (e.g Burrows, 1992; Lowe, 1992), but ethical reflectiveness and philosophical analysis of all the issues should lead to a clearer understanding of the problems and stronger possibilities for moral interventions.

The practitioner–client relationship

Deterioration in the therapeutic relationship would seem to be a likely result when a client has been restrained or medicated against his/her wishes as a result of assaultive behaviour. The consequences of damage to the caring relationship can be loss of trust, and fear and anxiety for both carer and client. But the client's violent behaviour may be part of the testing out of staff, a response to care rather than control (Breakwell, 1989). Staff must be aware of such testing out behaviours but also aware when aggression may develop beyond staff members' control and become dangerous.

For the client the initial mental health problem is compounded by the loss of personal control and limited self-determination. The staff member maintains control on behalf of the organisation and ultimately society. But the client may find a sense of control through aggression and therefore repeat the behaviours to gain some degree of self-determination. When dealing with clients seeking gains in this manner, it is the control and power that are invested in the practitioner that cause discomfort and anxiety for many members of staff. The conflicts arising may result in some staff becoming 'burnt out' and apathetic; this can lead to long-term sickness. The feeling of loss of power, when confronted with a violent client, may also be difficult for practitioners to deal with:

> "One social worker after an attack explained: 'I felt patronised and humiliated, as though my superior position as a social worker has gone. I didn't feel angry or even hurt. I felt – I am in the caring role and look what happened'." (Breakwell, 1989)

Strong emotions and distress felt by many members of staff as a result of caring for assaultive clients are hard to resolve – debriefing counselling, peer and management support are essential but also staff must be given permission to show their emotions – to 'put a brave face on' is not always the most helpful thing to do. The provision of post-incident support is discussed in greater detail in Chapter 7. Staff should be taught how to deal with their own emotional reactions as well as understanding how anger can affect the client's thought processes. For the client faulty cognitions can cause information to be processed incorrectly, resulting in an immediate failure to follow instructions and increasing the likelihood of interpretative bias, so that he/she may fail to learn from the aggressive incident but rely on stereotypical interpretations of the reasons for the anger at the root of the incident.

In the therapeutic relationship, after an aggressive incident, trust must be regained, respect and dignity maintained, information given to allow a more equal relationship and new goals of care identified and negotiated to allow the client to work with the practitioner without losing personal control. Some control, through limit setting, may need to be agreed in the process of negotiation, to provide safe boundaries for the client's behaviour:

> "Setting limits involves an ability to be firm and to know when to exert control. It refers to the imposition of necessary and specific constraints upon behaviour." (Lowe, 1992)

Control of violence as the organisational norm

Case example 8.3

> Jo, a new nursing assistant on an acute admission ward in a large hospital, was faced with Michael, a large, often aggressive patient, threatening to hit him – he called over the other nursing assistant, Frank, but managed on his own to calm Michael down. The other staff, especially Frank, commented afterwards "It's the last time I'll come over . . . next time you need help you'll see if we're there to back you up". Jo felt that he was different from the others and would not get help if a patient attacked him. He felt he would have to conform to being hard like the others or he would be on his own.

Repeated exposures to aggression and violence in any organisation or institution may have unforeseen effects on the therapeutic milieu. The staff must be aware of norms and values that they may be socialised into which may militate against therapy and prevention of violence. If the prevalent ideology is based on the medical model where 'cure' rather than 'care' is valued and client behaviours, especially assaultive behaviours, are, at times, seen as symptoms of an illness rather than as a result of environmental factors such as lack of personal space, then the resulting norms and staff behaviours may reflect an authoritarian and inflexible model of care, in which blanket security policies stifle individualised care.

Research carried out in the USA (Morrison, 1990) showed that unqualified members of staff were socialised by other staff members into using physical methods of restraint rather than verbal therapeutic methods, and that control was enforced through attitudes of toughness and confrontation with group pressure to conform to this culture. The result of this 'machismo' among those who interacted most with the clients, combined with emphasis on rules and inflexible staff attitudes, was an increase of violent behaviour. When staff:client ratios were increased violence surprisingly increased because there was more chances of stressful staff–client interactions. The increased rate of violent behaviours often found at hand-overs/shift changes supports these findings. Similar values and norms have unfortunately been found in the UK too:

> "We believe that a number of practices are somewhat controlling and encourage defensive behaviours. Impoverished and closed environments, routines associated with total institutionalisation, over-reliance on rules, symbols and security all serve to reinforce a devalued image and culture." (Blom-Cooper Report; Department of Health, 1992)

In organisations where male members of staff predominate at all levels this culture of 'machismo' is more likely to be prevalent and values associated with caring be dismissed as 'soft'. Female staff may overcompensate in this atmosphere of toughness, in institutions where challenging, self-injurious and violent behaviours are frequently encountered, by tending to act at least as tough as their male colleagues.

Again, the constraints of security impinging on the primary goal of therapeutic, humanistic care must be addressed. Empowerment of clients, independent advocacy services and flexibility of management rather than rigid structures will counteract values of control and power.

Staff induction programmes must include, for all levels (and for bank/agency nurses), training on verbal de-escalation and other therapeutic techniques as well as control and restraint methods. There must be a culture and structure of clinical supervision to enhance good practices and raise awareness of therapeutic interventions, and there should be a mix of levels and expertise of staff in clinical areas.

Members of staff should also be recognised for therapeutic initiatives in their 'individual performance reviews', and they should be valued by peers, managers and other disciplines. Members of staff must also have the freedom to report unethical behaviour and to question rigid or over-harsh rules. Above all, an organisational value system of cooperation within care would result in decreasing the traditions of toughness.

The use of control and restraint when the carer is the target of violence

Although the legal case for self-defence may be clear, the professional ethics of self-defence are not explicit. The *Code of Professional Conduct* of the UK Central Council for Nurses, Midwives and Health Visitors (1992) stresses that the actions of nurses must not be detrimental to their clients, so that when a nurse is threatened or assaulted by a client to whom a duty to care exists, they are then placed in the dilemma of constraining the client's autonomy and self-determined actions in order to preserve the carer's own safety and self-interest.

If practitioners have unsuccessfully tried other preventive measures and breakaway techniques, however, they may justify measures of self-defence as protecting other clients, both in the immediate situation if they are at risk of further harm, and in the longer term if, by preventing injury to themselves which would entail sick leave, they are therefore more able to give quality of care to the other clients.

In reality, practitioners are often faced with sanctions by management concerning the use of self-defence and therefore become anxious and more unwilling to take therapeutic risks. The result is then increased sickness rates, with further deterioration of care or more control in care with less choice and self-determination for clients. Use of self-defence may be seen by some as a failure to use alternative strategies or as unjustifiable use of control and power over vulnerable people; but when staff have adequate preparation for the possibility of assault, including training and guidance from managers, where other interventions have actively been attempted and when restraint techniques are used for the shortest possible time, then no sense of victimisation or guilt should be implied. Management has a duty to provide safety at work for employees, and attempts to prevent or sanction the use of appropriate self-defence techniques could be held as negligence in the duty of management to prevent harm to staff.

Whose responsibility is it to assist assaultive clients?

Outside of the therapeutic relationship, or the institutional health and social service structures, there exists no general duty to care imposed upon the practitioner, or indeed citizens in general. If, for example, a nurse in a hospital ward finds that a patient while taking a bath has slipped under the water and is drowning there is a clear responsibility upon the nurse to attempt to rescue the patient – not to do so would be negligent. If, though, on the journey home from work the nurse encounters a stranger drowning in a river there is no requirement in law for the nurse to attempt a rescue.

This chapter, however, assumes as a starting point that the readers of this book work within health care or social care relationships and in these circumstances the duty to care is axiomatic. With regard to the client who is over-assertive, aggressive or assaultive the same duty of care exists: it is not usurped by the client's behaviour, however unreasonable.

One aspect of the therapeutic relationship that is often under-represented is the notion that the client, as well as being in the patient's role, has clear responsibilities within the therapeutic relationship, and that all citizens, and most especially mentally disordered citizens, must be encouraged to exercise their responsibilities as well as their rights. Responsibilities of the citizen within a society are subject to cultural variation and to some extent may be distilled from statute. Regarding English law and society, Baker (1982) asserts that "Absolute freedom does not exist, since one man's right is another man's duty".

The area of negligence, that is failure to exercise the duty to care, is under constant change and revision, although some comfort is available to the practitioner by section 139 of the Mental Health Act 1983 (for England and Wales), which states that persons acting in pursuance of the Act would not normally be liable "unless the act was done in bad faith or without reasonable care"; Jones (1988) expounds a further explanation of this section and Underwood (1985) provides an interesting review of the law pertaining to professional negligence.

Case example 8.4

John was admitted to a general hospital psychiatric ward and was diagnosed as having an acute organic brain disorder (he had been given penicillin the day before by his general practitioner for a streptococcal throat infection). John was visually hallucinating, occasionally striking out at the air and shouting at 'faces' that he could see. The registrar, checking his patients before leaving for home, went to see John – who, presumably mistaking the registrar for a 'face' struck out at the registrar and then commenced to squeeze him about the throat. The registrar was rescued by patients and staff.

Once it has been established that a client has clarity of thought and is capable of making informed choices it would be reasonable to expect that person to respect the rights of the carer to maintain his/her integrity and to operate within the boundaries of the therapeutic relationship – where the parameters of a health care relationship are unclear, contracts may have to be considered. It was clear to all that John, while temporarily unbalanced, was not capable at that time of making an informed choice to strangle the registrar.

Case example 8.5

On the same unit, but within a different ward, was Julie, who had had frequent admissions to the unit. Julie was 23 years old and was described as being 'inadequate' and as having psychopathic tendencies: she would take measured overdoses of prescribed medication when wishing to be admitted to hospital; frequently was assaultive when drunk; and occasionally committed petty crimes. Finally, the mental health team, unable to assist her to change some of her more unreasonable behaviours, and despite repeated negotiated contracts being set and then broken by Julie, decided that she should not in future be admitted to the hospital ward but would instead be offered support on a day-care basis, as appropriate. Upon hearing this Julie walked out of the ward and began to smash windows in the hospital corridor. The staff decided that Julie should be reported to the police for these criminal acts as she was in control of her actions and was failing to exercise a reasonable amount of responsibility.

For those who work in institutional settings such as hospitals, health centres, residential homes and the like, there also exists a legal imperative upon the managers of the institution to ensure the health and safety of persons within that environment (Mitchell, 1975; Barrett & Howells, 1993). The Department of Health and Social Security (DHSS) issued a health circular in 1976 (HC 76/11) that instructed its recipients to prepare guidance for all staff members on care and management of the violent or potentially violent individual. The DHSS had become concerned about the apparent increase in the incidence of violence within the health service and the patchy response to addressing issues concerning the environment of care and the appropriate preparation of staff to care for assaultive people.

In a resource-restricted health and social service system there will always be tensions about how resources might best be used and so the amount of preparation in terms of training and education offered to staff on a variety of issues will be locally determined. Ways of prioritising training are discussed in Chapter 6. As a minimum, however, all staff should be issued with written guidelines on caring for assaultive clients, and where assaults by clients or others are not uncommon it would be reasonable for further resources, perhaps in the form of personal attack alarms (or in the community radios/pagers) to be allocated, and for staff to receive training in the management of commoner incidents.

Indeed, in a number of units where physical attack is frequent, for example inner-city casualty departments and acute psychiatric units, the managers would be remiss in not addressing this agenda. Once the employee has been given guidance, in whatever form, the onus is upon him/her to act within the guidance – otherwise the legal indemnity provided by the employer in case of client litigation at a later date may be lost (Tarbuck, 1992).

What actions are legally permissible should a carer be attacked?

According to Cremona (1989) the criminal law of assault "is often illogical both in content and terminology, and the whole area, including sexual assaults, is ready for reform". Smith & Hogan (1988) agree that the law contains some inconsistencies and anomalies. They do go on to state, however, that:

> "The general principle . . . is that the law allows such force as is reasonable in the circumstances of the particular case . . .what is reasonable [is] to be judged in the light of the circumstances as the accused believed them to be, whether reasonably or not."

This principle is based upon section 3(1) of the Criminal Law Act 1967, which permits:

> "Such force as is reasonable in the circumstances in the prevention of crime, or in effecting or assisting in the lawful arrest of offenders or of persons unlawfully at large."

While lawyers may care to debate and argue over the legal interpretation of various aspects of the criminal law and associated aspects of common law, there does appear to be a legal 'rock' upon which the practitioner might care to set down a marker. While this tenet of 'reasonable force' may provide some comfort to staff in an increasingly violent and litigation-minded society, the mental health practitioner must also be concerned about the maintenance of a therapeutic relationship after an incident has occurred – which, even during the event, the enlightened practitioner will remain aware of. Because of this it is of the utmost importance that a practitioner's response is reasonable in the circumstances so that once the assaultive person is calm it may then be possible to appeal to a sense of fair play and minimise the damage to the therapeutic relationship. Dealing with the client at the end of an aggressive incident is dealt with in more detail in Chapter 4.

Case example 8.5

Bill was resident in a medium-secure setting, having agreed to reside there for treatment of a psychotic illness during which his paranoid delusions had caused him to attack a neighbour. Bill believed at the time of the assault that the neighbour had been interfering with his electricity supply (this was not the case). Bill had been in the unit for five months and was stabilising well on antipsychotic medication and had commenced day trips back into the community. While out on a day trip Bill had a chance meeting with an ex-girlfriend and she and Bill had spent the afternoon together. Bill was an hour late returning to the unit and Bill's primary nurse approached him for details of his unpunctuality. Bill rounded on the nurse in a verbal tirade full of invective and expletives. The primary nurse, surprised by this apparent change in character and taken aback by the ferociousness of the verbal assault, suggested that Bill might like to rest in his room for ten minutes. Bill stormed past the primary nurse, pushing him violently into the wall using his shoulder, and the nurse's arm caught the sharp corner of a picture frame; Bill disappeared into his room. After ten minutes the primary nurse entered Bill's room, along with the registrar, to enquire what had occurred. Bill, with a cigarette and a cup of tea, said that the primary nurse had been annoying him and that the day's activities were none of their concern. Not only Bill's demeanour but also his physical appearance had changed; his pupils were dilated and his speech slightly slurred – both carers suspected that Bill had been taking alcohol or other substances that were now reacting with his antipsychotic medication. After a further hour, Bill was a little more amenable to cooperation and agreed to supply a sample of urine for testing for drugs, volunteering that he had spent the afternoon with an ex-girlfriend and had taken four blue tablets that his acquaintance had advised would bring Bill some peace. The day following the incident Bill was profusely apologetic to the primary nurse both for the verbal altercation and for pushing him into the wall. The primary nurse accepted Bill's apology, believing his actions to be the result of intoxication and therefore that Bill was not in total control of himself. Bill had shown genuine remorse for his actions and was probably concerned about the effects of his temporary lapse upon his future care plan. The nurse believed that incident could be used to build the trust and mutual respect characteristic of the therapeutic relationship, as well as being a learning experience for Bill.

What practical guidance is available on caring for assaultive clients?

The *Code of Practice Mental Health Act 1983* (Department of Health and Welsh Office, 1993) represents a guide to good practice in the affairs of detained mentally disordered people. Similar guidance is available in other parts of the UK.

The *Code* does not impose legal duties on mental health practitioners; however, it does indicate that "failure to follow the *Code* could be referred to in evidence in legal proceedings". The *Code* affirms, and builds upon the movement towards an enlightened approach to the provision of mental health services in which clients are respected for themselves as unique individuals; cultural attributes and diversity are acknowledged; self-determination and responsibility are encouraged; and services offered are the least restrictive practicable for that individual.

Section 18 of the *Code* concerns patients presenting particular management problems and gives guidance upon precursors to aggression and their prevention; restraint; medication; seclusion; locking doors and wards; observation of patients; and the deprivation of day-time clothing. Although issues of restraint and seclusion appear in the same section of the *Code* it must not be assumed that there is an automatic association between the two.

Modern techniques of physical restraint mean that clients may be held in a safe manner (i.e. under control but not in pain) for extended periods of time, which enables the practitioners to experiment with less socially isolating forms of de-escalation and to release the holds as clients resume their own locus of control. Both the Blom-Cooper Report (Department of Health, 1992) and Topping-Morris (1993) suggest that the use of seclusion should ultimately become redundant and as this captures the gist of contemporary thought on the matter the use of seclusion must be considered as a matter of extreme gravity and only for as short time as is possible. Indeed, its use can only be accepted in situations where patients are persisting with violent behaviour (despite repeated and enduring non-physical attempts to de-escalate the tension), and where less socially isolating management techniques have proved ineffective.

All mental health staff in England and Wales are expected to be conversant with the principles and guidance within the *Code*, and sections 18.5 and 18.6 of the *Code* give guidance about avoiding aggressive incidents which include:

(a) good communications with patients and access for patients to external communications media
(b) acknowledgement of personal space and privacy requirements
(c) provision of a programme of therapeutic activities that are suited to individuals' needs
(d) monitoring of patient mix and appropriate staff skills mix via training

(e) access to an equitable and efficient patients' complaints procedure.

Further and more detailed guidance on the prevention and avoidance of violence can be found in the works of Owen & Ashcroft (1985) and Ritter (1989), as well as in other parts of this volume.

Sections 18.10 and 18.11 of the *Code* indicate appropriate actions for institutionally based staff to take when faced with an episode of assaultive behaviour. For future editions of the *Code* it would be desirable for these sections to be expanded so that guidance may be given to non-institutional workers, as they cannot rely upon help being immediately available. There is evidence that these particular groups of mental health workers do face aggression (e.g. Health and Safety Commission, 1987) and it is likely that, as clients with challenging behaviours or those who are non-compliant with treatment are placed in the community, the incidence of aggression will escalate.

Conclusions

Staff faced with ethical dilemmas when caring for assaultive clients must maintain, as a core therapeutic objective, the ideal of restoring to the client her/his autonomy. This will take the form of freedom of choice and self-determination of behaviour as soon as is possible through using the least restrictive forms of intervention; autonomy will be enhanced by giving information and resting care and responsibility with the client rather than control or retribution being visited upon the client from a misguided paternalistic standpoint. The healthy therapeutic relationship with an assaultive client is dynamic and responsive; it is denoted by calculated therapeutic risk taking, limit setting and negotiation.

The legal perspectives concerning dealing with the assaultive client are relatively straightforward – provided the carer acts in good faith and with reasonable care he/she should not fall foul of the law. Where a carer is faced with an assaultive client his/her actions should be reasonable within the circumstances and be based upon the avoidance of physical contact; where the scenario has become physical the carer should use only the minimal force necessary for the minimal amount of time to bring the physical encounter to an end. Employees are expected to act consistently with the training they have received and in accord with their employer's policy and guidelines.

Summary points

- Paternalistic actions to prevent harm (however well intentioned) always entail some risk to the client's autonomy.
- Any actions taken by any carer should be reasonable within the circumstances in which the action is taken.
- The carer must ensure that any physical interventions used to control a situation are used for the shortest possible time, and that any physical force being used is kept to the absolute minimum.
- The carer must attempt to create more self-determination for the constrained individual by giving explanations and information; enabling the individual to resume control of him-/herself as soon as possible; and re-negotiating the care after the incident.
- Mentally disordered persons must not only be empowered to exercise their rights but also must be encouraged to exercise their responsibilities as citizens.
- Organisational values of caring for clients as individuals, flexibility, recognition of good practices and a climate of collaborative care will enhance the therapeutic milieu and minimise the potential for aggressive or violent situations to occur.
- Carers have needs for safety in their clinical areas that must be recognised: training in the management of the environment; verbal de-escalation of aggressive situations, and in self-defence techniques (such as breakaway techniques) will reduce the carer's anxiety levels and lead to increased confidence.

Where assaultive behaviours are not uncommon within the workplace the employer has a clear responsibility to provide the resources necessary to make the environment of care as safe as is reasonably practicable – this will include education and training for all members of staff who have contact with assaultive clients. The preparation and development of staff members must entail clinical supervision, opportunities for reflective practice (e.g. sharing personal decisions with peers in order to validate intuitive responses) and ethical and legal awareness, alongside the more traditional forms of education and training in caring for the assaultive client.

Members of staff who feel adequately prepared and informed will have confidence and the knowledge that it is possible to offer care to assaultive clients in a moral way, and within legally acceptable parameters. This preparation and information will empower the carer to enjoy the therapeutic relationship with these most challenging of individuals.

References

ATKINSON, J. (1991) Autonomy and mental health. In *Ethical Issues in Mental Health* (eds P. Barker & S. Baldwin). pp 103–106. London: Chapman & Hall.

BAKER, N. L. (1982) *The Law and the Individual.* Plymouth: Mcdonald & Evans.

BARRETT, R. & HOWELLS, R. (1993) *Health and Safety Law M+E Handbook.* London: Pitman.

BREAKWELL, G. (1989) *Facing Physical Violence.* London: BPS Books.

BURROWS, S. (1991) The special hospital nurse and the dilemma of therapeutic custody. *Journal of Advances in Health and Nursing Care,* 1, 21–28.

CREMONA, M. (1989) *Criminal Law.* Basingstoke: Macmillan Education.

DEPARTMENT OF HEALTH AND SOCIAL SECURITY (1976) Care of the Violent or Potentially Violent Individual, Health Circular 1976/11. London: Department of Health and Social Security.

DEPARTMENT OF HEALTH & SPECIAL HOSPITALS SERVICE AUTHORITY (1992) *Report of the Committee of Inquiry into Complaints about Ashworth Hospital. Blom-Cooper Report (Chairman: Sir Louis Blom-Cooper).* London: HMSO.

—— & WELSH OFFICE (1993) *Code of Practice Mental Health Act 1983.* London: HMSO.

ETH, S. & MILLS, M. (1990) Treating patients who threaten violence. In *Ethical Practice in Psychiatry and the Law,* vol. 7. (eds R. Rosner & R. Weinstock). New York : Plenum Press.

HEALTH AND SAFETY EXECUTIVE (1989) *Violence to Staff,* IND(G) 1\89 M100. London: HMSO.

HOGGETT, B. (1990) *Mental Health Law* (3rd edn). London: Sweet & Maxwell.

JONES, R. (1988) *Mental Health Act Manual* (2nd edn). London: Sweet & Maxwell.

LOWE, T. (1992) Characteristics of effective nursing interventions in the management of challenging behaviours. *Journal of Advanced Nursing,* 17, 1226–1232.

MITCHELL, E. (1975) *The Employer's Guide to the Law on Health, Safety and Welfare at Work.* London: Business Books.

MORRISON, E. (1990) The tradition of toughness *IMAGE: Journal of Nursing Scholarship,* 22, 1.

OWEN, R. G. & ASHCROFT, J. B. (1985) *Violence: A Guide for the Caring Professions.* Beckenham: Croom Helm.

RITTER, S. (1989) *Bethlem Royal and Maudsley Hospital : Manual of Clinical Psychiatric Nursing Principles and Procedures.* London: Harper & Row.

SEEDHOUSE, D. (1989) *Ethics – The Heart of Health Care.* London: Wiley.

SMITH, J. C. & HOGAN, B. (1988) *Criminal Law* (6th edn). London: Butterworths.

SPECIAL HOSPITALS SERVICE AUTHORITY (1993) *The Committee of Inquiry into the Death at Broadmoor Hospital of Orville Blackwood and a Review of the Deaths of Two Other Afro-Caribbean Patients: Big, Black and Dangerous?* London: SHSA.

TARBUCK, P. (1992) Use and abuse of control and restraint. *Nursing Standard,* 6, 30–32.

TOPPING-MORRIS, B. (1993) *Guidance upon Seclusion.* London: Royal College of Nursing.

UNDERWOOD, A. (ed.) (1985) *Underwood and Holt's Professional Negligence.* London: Fourmat.

UNITED KINGDOM CENTRAL COUNCIL FOR NURSES, MIDWIVES AND HEALTH VISITORS (1992) *Code of Professional Conduct* (3rd edn). London: UKCC.

Index

Compiled by CAROLINE SHEARD